AF480631

MATTHEW SAUNDERS

Normal: A Lifetime of Disabilities, Addictions and Diagnoses

Contents

II   My Chosen Life

III   Reflections

Acknowledgments

NORMAL is dedicated to everyone mentioned in this book. The life that I have been blessed to live would not be possible without all the people that shared these experiences with me.

To my beautiful wife, Christina and our amazing children, Alex, Olivia and Jacob—I'm not entirely sure how I would be here today without you. I love you more than words can express, and I cherish every moment we have together.

To my sister, Kelly. You have been the one constant since the day I was born, loving me unconditionally and always being there for me and my family. You've been my rock throughout everything. My love for you is endless.

There are also people who may not find their names woven into these chapters, but whose presence shaped this journey just as much. Family and friends who checked in without needing updates. Coworkers who quietly carried the load when I couldn't. Neighbors who showed up with food, rides, or a simple "thinking of you." People like my brother-in-law Dan, Liz & Gil, Anna, Derek and my entire Badger Basketball Family—they never asked for recognition and never needed it. If you're reading this and wondering whether you're included here—if you sat with us, laughed with us, prayed for us, or simply stayed when things got hard—know this: you mattered more than you'll ever realize, and this book carries your fingerprints too.

Lastly, I want to acknowledge the doctors, nurses, and staff at Froedtert & the Medical College of Wisconsin and Moffitt Cancer Center. Over the years, these places became more than hospitals. They are where fear was met with calm, where hard news was delivered with compassion, and where my family and I were treated as people — not just patients. The care I have received goes far beyond medicine, and the humanity shown to us during some of our hardest moments will stay with me for the rest of my life.

Disclaimer

This story is deeply personal. In sharing it, I've taken care to protect the identities of those who may not have chosen to tell their own stories publicly. Names and identifying details have been changed to protect the privacy of certain individuals.

Foreword

by Kelly Saunders

I have Mom's brown eyes - flecked with hazel, sunken into a Celtic brow that makes people assume I am irritated or angry when I'm not. Really, they are her father's eyes, our grandfather Aloysius, who neither of us met but who loomed large in childhood stories. You have Dad's eyes, the Saunders tourmaline blue, that can shift almost translucent in a defining rim of deep navy, tucked safely behind long curled lashes that proved the envy of our many aunts.

Those blue eyes saved you, as the recycled childhood story revealed early on during a ridiculous backyard proposition, prompted by older siblings feeling crowded for attention and space: if Mom and Dad had to give up one of their four children, we declared, it had to be you. Adam was first born and therefore safe, my protection was a complicated status of only girl, and Andrew held special magic that only a 23rd chromosome provides. It was decided. But you fervently contended through your tears that you also had to stay in the family because you were the only child with blue eyes.

Now I can easily see the inheritance of our family when I look at you, a winding map of brotherhood, loyalty, heartache and love. We labeled you "the Golden Child" early on, for you seemed to have won Dad's heart in a unique way, a closeness

Adam and I craved but didn't consistently find. Mom agreed but asserted that it came from almost losing you before you were born - her late pregnancy hemorrhage, the doctor's contention that you hadn't survived it, their joy at your birth because you were absolutely perfect - a gift from God.

We carry the whole family in these stories that live freely in my chaotic mind and often shift, with embellishment or fact checks, depending on the teller. It's hard to discern which stories hold the most truth or desired evidence that we once grew up in a seemingly happy family. Sure, there are photographs to corroborate a bit of normalcy, though they are far and few between, ancient handheld relics from a Disney vacation or RV road trip to national parks. The settings shift quickly over time, from church sacristy to doughnut shop, school gymnasiums and gas stations, a river parkway, a campus, way too many hospitals. I sometimes envy the ease at which you'll jump into any photo being taken when I've worked to avoid them. They always seem too static or curated, impossible to capture anything close to all that is alive in that moment. I know with certainty that no photograph, no lines clumsily written by my tired hands, can capture all of your indomitable spirit.

My highlight reel is filled with beginnings, untouched by detours and complications, with you embracing adventure and possibility with wide open arms. I see you and Dan Gaus running up the porch steps of my first college apartment, eager high school buddies anxious to join every bit of revelry before your first Pearl Jam concert. And I could probably sketch the instant you thrust open the maternity room doors of St. Joseph's hospital at the exact moment I arrived, locking eyes for just a split second before a quick pivot to the crowded waiting room for your announcement that Alex had arrived. Often, I see you in motion, walking quickly toward me during a sunrise layover at Sea-Tac airport for a handoff of frosted cookies before your flight home from a basketball tournament or grabbing my hand to jump off the Park City shuttle bus and race to the front of the ticket line at the Sundance premiere of a Beastie Boys documentary. I see you sprinting across the parking lot of Miller Park to hug me home from my Ghana adventures before your GMR Rock Star event or weaving quickly through proud parents at the elementary school science fair to say hello. You leading us from a Sussex baseball diamond, your arms filled with equipment that you dropped to the gravel parking lot to revel in the news that Ella was coming. Countless times you scooped my girl up in later years, greeting her every entry with an enthusiastic EB! and generous smile.

There are also those worn-out stories of our youth, repurposed into a familiar refrain. You freezing your tongue on the front yard flagpole to fulfill a dare, the nicotine-hazed Yahtzee games at Grandma's kitchen table, our pride at carrying Aunt Pearl's handwritten note to pick up her Virginia Slim Menthol cigarettes at Court Drugs, my dramatic indignation when you and Adam snatched my bowl of fresh cookie dough from my hands. Stories of Andrew's escapades to the Augustine's basketball hoop or his solo trek from your dorm to the UW Field House to bring candy bars to Stu Jackson. Late-night Spanish homework faxed from Seattle to Madison within hours of a due date. The fateful day Chrissie stopped into Dad's gas station. Perhaps we rewind these scenes out of nostalgia or to evoke a laugh with close cousins and old friends - and maybe we don't let them go because so much of what came after those moments is way too hard.

Most of the time, our painful B-roll stays hidden, though the consequences exist in sharp relief. I try to keep its roots in a fuzzy fast forward - a twisted knee injury on an old ball field, too many painkillers, a daytime arrest and then another, and another. Mom's spiteful refusal to pull our family back together. Someday I hope to edit any reminder of Jake's birthday dinner when we stood listening to her accusations in your kitchen, knowing that our family was broken. You knew there were kids to protect, regardless of how awful it became. I regret how long it took me to leave the mess after a series of futile attempts to convince Mom of addiction's demands, to give Andrew something normal, to help Dad escape, too.

It seemed impossible, too, that our sorrow would grow one January evening when you called me to share your diagnosis as I sat in the grocery store parking lot with a warm rotisserie chicken in my hands. You had cancer, not the treatable, temporary bout I'd recently experienced but serious and life altering, the kind that brings extensive surgery and treatment, pain and seismic shifts for your young family. The onslaught of appointments and lab work, second opinions, testing and tedious waits.

However stacked your deck became, it was always crystal clear (still is) that for you, love is action, a forward-looking generous motion, powerful and practiced deeply to garner strength and hope. Whatever details unfolded about your body, your heart was beating for Chrissie, Alex, Olivia, Jake. After your first surgery, I stood with Chrissie in a long hospital corridor trying to decipher what, if anything, we were to do next to avoid despair, but we were speechless. I left to find Dad praying his rosary in the twilight, still sitting in the waiting room chair he found before sunrise, still trying to reconcile how any of this could be happening to his beautiful boy. By then, Dad's eyes did most of his communicating since he struggled so much to find his words. What were we to do for your kids, so full of light, carrying those blue eyes, your infectious humor and sense of wonder, toothy smiles and lanky limbs, a whole roster of stories yet to be told? What we would do, you insisted, is stop wringing our hands and instead, wield hope like an axe, breaking down doors in this emergency.

And so we did. I bore witness to your superhuman efforts to get well without complaint, never losing your signature wit and smile. Hope was finally brimming, so much so that I actually agreed to shoot a commercial for the new cancer center so you could share your story. Strangers and old friends alike got to see for themselves your desire to live with intention, to help others. The sucker punch that followed wasn't just confounding, it extinguished our momentary reprieve, the only pinprick of solace that Dad never had to know your cancer returned. And yet again, you would not let us be suffocated by that news. There were things to do and moves to be made.

The hardest of those tasks was saying goodbye to Dad, with the full understanding that the end of his time on earth was nothing less than a nightmare. As we navigated the rapid deterioration of his mind and the indignities of losing his once strong and vital body, we also knew that he would not want us to lose time to sorrow. When we visited him on his 80th birthday, a once towering father now tiny in child's pose, you brought him a brightly colored cupcake and laughed with him as he devoured all the thick frosting. He said only one word that day - your name - the last one I heard him say before I held his hand as he died not two months later. It's an unsolvable riddle that even then, Mom refused to relent her spite but none of that mattered anymore. When you stood at the funeral pulpit to honor him before all who loved him at St. Margaret Mary, palpable with childhood memories, you easily made visible his love for us, his pride in his family, and the legacy you carry forward.

Part of that legacy lives here, for Dad was a storyteller just like our Gramps. Regardless of how many losses we tallied, we know stories can save us, too. Here's one of my favorites, sparked from a single day in Pittsburgh: We were so elated that Wisconsin had made it to the NCAA basketball tournament, only their second bid in 56 years. You'd graduate from college that spring, just before your fall wedding but for now, you'd be on that Badger bench. My Seattle friends thought it was crazy that I'd fly across the country for a basketball game with my brothers, but they didn't get it. It wasn't something to miss. When Texas ran away with the game from the beginning and blew out Wisconsin's dreams for another round so completely, you came to the stands from the locker room, and we sat for just a moment silent as the arena cleared. Boy, we were sad. Devastated, stunned. That was the ending, or so we thought, but it wasn't really. We celebrated all night in Pittsburgh, an unfamiliar city but exactly the right place, surrounded by so many friends, players, fans, family. It was pure joy.

These days, I look more like Mom, and you look more like Dad than ever. But in my dreams, we're still young and impatient, heading back to the Columbia River for an afternoon of whitewater rafting or racing through rows of a concert venue with Ami to hear Soundgarden play again. We march with a crowd of drunken Badger fans, lifted from 17 S.

Randall to State Street, a chain of arms locked while singing *Varsity* and celebrating our wins.

Mostly, though, I see you as I've always seen you, entirely free of disease, setting off to your next adventure, arms and eyes wide open, that mischievous grin gathering the people you love, relentlessly dreaming. A life to live without any wasted moments - golden.

Introduction

Normal *[nawr-muhl]:*

Adjective

Conforming to the standard or the common type; usual; not abnormal; regular; natural.

It's such a simple word and most people assume they know what it means, but no one truly knows *normal*. I would venture to guess that if asked, 100 out of 100 would have at least one aspect of their lives that is not *normal*—it's just not that simple.

This book is for those that have accepted their lives as *normal*, knowing deep down that abnormal is actually the norm, but it's also for those that need help understanding that what they have in life is theirs to appreciate, regardless of the circumstances. No one has a perfect life, at least not by society's standards, but we can love the life we have, no matter what the universe throws at us.

I guess, the point is that once you've accepted your life for what it is, it becomes your *normal*, and finding the positives in all that you have is the first step towards living your life to the fullest extent—accepting the cards you've been dealt and making the most out of it. You can strive for more while still having a deep appreciation for what you hold.

I wish everyone that takes the time to read this the very best. My purpose in drafting this book is to show the world that your life doesn't have to be a scripted fairy tale at every turn to truly enjoy yourself. I have navigated through many difficult situations in my life but have found the positives in each one to help me appreciate what's really important.

I

My Given Life

CHAPTER 1: I'm Dying

I'm dying. Not all at once. Not dramatically. Not in the way people imagine when they hear that word. But I am living with the knowledge that something inside my body is actively working to end my life. And once you know that, dying stops being a distant idea. It becomes something you feel. Something you carry. Something that changes how you move through the world.

In January of 2016, I sat silently in a noisy conference room as a dozen coworkers talked over each other, brainstorming our next big idea. The energy in the room was loud and confident, ideas bouncing across the large oval table, but I felt strangely removed from it all—like I was the only one actually sitting there. I knew a call was coming. I didn't know exactly when it would come, or what it would say, only that it could change everything. And then it happened, my phone began to buzz. A number I didn't recognize, but a call I needed to answer. My heart raced as I picked up the phone and quietly snuck out of the room. The rest is a bit of a blur. The short walk to find some sort of privacy in my cubicle was all the time the doctor needed to tell me the news—*you have cancer.* I sat slumped in my office chair, trying desperately to process the news—once again feeling alone and helpless.

In the subsequent months, I would learn that I had Stage III colorectal cancer, along with a malignant neuroendocrine tumor on my pancreas. I endured surgeries, chemotherapy, and radiation—the whole exhausting, demoralizing cycle of treatment. Somehow, I made it through. I rang the bell. I looked forward to brighter days ahead.

The subsequent five years weren't without challenges. I lived with the long-term effects of cancer and its treatment—side effects that doctors prepare you for medically but not emotionally. But I survived. And I made it to what they call your "cure date": June 21, 2021. Five years from when the doctors surgically removed the cancer from my body. A day that I had circled, prayed for, visualized.

My wife, Christina, and I celebrated that milestone the way you commemorate a hard-earned victory. We had traveled out west to share this moment with our best friends. A celebratory dinner in downtown Colorado Springs. Good food, stiff drinks and plenty of hugs. It felt like hope. It felt like breathing again. For the first time in years, I thought I could maybe stop looking over my shoulder. We all basked in the glory of what we thought was a long-overdue and well-deserved triumph.

Unfortunately, the victory was short-lived, as just a month later, I had an appointment that would undo it all. One last follow up scan to ensure I was finally in the clear, but something wasn't right. There were concerning spots on my images that gave my care team cause for trepidation. The pancreas specialist who had removed the small neuroendocrine tumor in 2016 was called in to consult. We sat nervously in the lobby, surrounded by a room full of patients doing the exact same thing, holding onto each other's hands, as well as hope, waiting for news. We were called into the tiny, sterile office where we were greeted by a small army of medical professionals, and in that moment, I think we already knew what we were about to hear. The neuroendocrine tumor, the one we were told five years ago we shouldn't have to worry about, had metastasized. My doctors had found twelve lesions (later updated to thirteen) on my liver. Malignant. The cancer was back and this time it was Stage IV.

Metastatic. Incurable. A death sentence without a date.

In some twisted way, it almost feels harder—not having a set date. If I were on death row, at least I'd have a calendar. I'd know the day and time I'd take my last breath. But with this diagnosis, there's no such clarity. Just an indefinite timeline of treatments, scans, faith, and setbacks. My doctors are doing everything they can to keep pushing that date further into the future. But make no mistake—death is the shadow that now walks beside me.

And yet, strangely and over time, I've found peace in that. I've reset. I've let go of the illusion that we ever really know how much time we have. I've become hyper-aware of how precious this life is—not in the cliché way you read on inspirational posters, but in the real, everyday kind of way. A warm hug from my kids. The smell of my wife's shampoo. Laughing at dumb TV shows together on the couch. These are the moments I've learned to savor.

Then there's the clinical side. My first round of treatment in 2016 was oral chemotherapy and 28 rounds of radiation. St. Patrick's Day marked the beginning. I wore my green tuxedo t-shirt that first day, clinging to some sense of humor, some sense of identity.

Every day, Christina would sit in the waiting room with me until they called my name. She'd give me a hug and wish me luck with tears running down her face, before retreating to her chair, still warm from the long wait. Radiation meant lying face down on a special table, surrounded by machines and nurses, with my backside exposed. One day, a nurse asked Christina if she wanted to join and observe the process. When the nurse asked if I was okay with Christina being in the room as I exposed my lower half prior to getting on the table, I joked, *"You all have seen my ass for weeks—my wife's seen it for years."* Laughter helped us stay human.

For my final day of radiation, I baked caramel cheesecake cups for the nurses, each one containing a letter that spelled out *"Thank You from the BOTTOM of My Heart."* It was corny, sweet, and entirely me.

Surgery that summer was brutal—eight hours long. When I woke up in that hospital bed, tubes and needles protruding from a dozen places on my body, I slowly tried to get my bearings. I hazily looked around, searching for Christina through the cloudy after-effects of the anesthesia. And then it hit me—I felt like I'd been run over by a truck. The pain in my abdomen was more intense than any morphine drip could mask. You definitely don't realize how much you use your core until someone slices through it and tells you not to cough, sneeze, lift or laugh for a while.

And then the ileostomy bag—by far the worst part. It changed everything. I mapped out porta-potties before Alex's baseball games. I lived in fear of sleeping wrong. For six months, I adjusted, managed, and survived. If given the option, I think I'd choose the six months of the grueling IV chemotherapy I endured in the fall and winter of 2016 over having that bag again.

There was a silver lining with the bag, however: I could eat dairy again (yes, I am lactose intolerant). Cheese, custard, ice cream—the foods I used to love but couldn't tolerate anymore. Still, if given the option, I'd never trade that joy for what I had to endure.

Since July of 2021, I have been following a new plan. Liver directed treatment every 28 days, along with endless scans and tests. And when the tumors began to progress in 2024, another major surgery, eerily similar to the procedure in 2016, to remove and ablate 11 of the 13 tumors. A success, for sure, but not a cure. There are certainly more tumors hiding in my liver, but as long as the two we can see don't progress and the unseen tumors don't present themselves, I can continue to fight on.

As the years pass, however, cancer is definitely taking a toll. I've been able to stay so mentally strong over the years, something that has helped me physically as well, but following this last procedure, I can tell I'm not the same. My mind is weaker and my body is absolutely suffering. But, the battle continues, and I won't give up hope.

Beyond treatment, there are the logistics. Being sick is a full-time job. Managing appointments, time off from work, insurance approvals. We've paid tens of thousands out of pocket—money that could've changed our future. I'm grateful for the help we've had, but sometimes the system feels stacked against us.

I've also learned how quickly it can all change. My life has become a masterclass in perspective.

There are five stages of grief: denial, anger, bargaining, depression, and acceptance. I've been through them all. My journey might not be unique, but it's deeply my own. Everyone processes these stages differently, and some don't experience every single one.

Christina, for example, hasn't, at least from what I can see, reached *acceptance*. We went through the *denial* phase together—clinging to optimism that somehow the doctors had it wrong. We held onto hope like a lifeline, waiting for some miraculous second opinion to wipe the board clean.

I was able to breeze past *anger*. There's no value in wasting energy on something that doesn't serve your recovery. Christina, though, still wrestles with it. She asks "why" often, knowing full well we'll never get an answer. It's not that she's angry at me—she's angry at what this disease has taken from us.

Bargaining was a short chapter. I know there's no value in "what ifs". Our focus needs to be forward—not dwelling on how cancer came to be part of our lives, but how we continue fighting. There's nothing that can be undone now, only what lies ahead.

Depression is one we both know too well. Mine comes in waves—sneaky and quiet. Just when I think I've escaped it, even for just a moment, a TV ad or a random line in a movie brings it roaring back. Cancer is inescapable in modern storytelling. It finds you, even when you're just trying to take a break and enjoy something light. Christina seems to shoulder her sadness differently. She doesn't break down often, but when she does, it's raw and honest. I've watched her cry as they call my name for treatment—each time it feels fresh again. That walk from the waiting room to the treatment room is always the same distance but somehow the weight with each step gets heavier each visit.

Acceptance came for me after my second diagnosis in 2021. I had time to reflect—time to find peace. If I had to leave this earth tomorrow, I could do so without regret. I'm proud to say that I've lived a full life already. I've experienced great love. I've raised three incredible kids with a woman who is stronger than I could ever put into words. Christina has not only been my partner in life, but my partner in this fight. She sits with me through every appointment, every infusion, every scan. And each time they call my name to go back for treatment, I see those eyes well up with tears—every single time. She tries to be strong, but I know what she's carrying. This isn't just my diagnosis. It's ours. So, for Christina? I don't think she'll ever fully let go of hope.

I can't say I haven't *grieved*. I absolutely have. I've had days where I allowed myself to fall apart—where I sobbed in the shower or lay in bed staring at the ceiling, wondering how I was going to tell my kids. Wondering how long I had before my wife would become a widow. But once that wave passes, what's left is something almost spiritual: gratitude. Not for the cancer, but for the way it's forced me to live more honestly, more openly, and more presently than I ever thought possible.

And then there are my kids: Alex, Olivia, and Jacob. I still remember sitting them down in 2016 to tell them the news the first time. They were so young. Too young to understand the weight of what I was saying. But they've grown up in a world where cancer is part of our family vocabulary. They've watched me lose weight and energy—but never hope. We celebrated my cure date, hugged a little tighter, and believed we were through the storm.

And then came the relapse. The shift. The gut punch. Another hard conversation. More uncertainty. Another steep hill to climb.

The kids have responded differently, however. Even on

the hardest days, the kids filled the house with noise—music, footsteps, laughter drifting down the hallway when I needed it most. I never saw them go through denial or anger. They don't know enough about how this started to bargain. They go straight to sadness. And fear. I know their greatest fear is losing their dad. And I carry that knowledge with me every day.

Children are resilient. They move toward acceptance more quickly than we do—maybe because their lives are still in motion. Maybe because, for them, this became one more thing to learn. In a strange way, this is part of their childhood story now.

What breaks my heart most isn't the fear of dying—it's the idea of not being there for the rest of their lives. Missing graduations. Weddings. Grandkids I'll never hold. It's the empty seat at the dinner table that haunts me.

But here's the thing: my children are stronger than they should have to be. They are compassionate, insightful, and spirited. And I truly believe that no matter what happens, they will take the love I've poured into them and carry it forward. Legacy is a strange word. For me, it's simple: Christina, Alex, Olivia, and Jacob. If they carry my love and strength into the world, that's more than enough. That's everything.

I don't pretend that this journey has been easy. There have been dark moments. But there have also been beautiful ones— the kind of beauty that only becomes visible when you're forced to confront what really matters. One moment stands out. At the Cathedral Basilica in St. Augustine, I sat in a pew while a college choir rehearsed. The soloist's voice filled the room, and suddenly I was crying. Not from fear, but from peace. That was the first time I realized I was ready. Not ready to go—but no longer afraid.

Together, Christina and I have let go of trivial things. We don't waste time on grudges. We speak openly, say *"I love you"* more often, and laugh even louder. And then, in the quiet, there's space to reflect. Sitting on our back patio watching the water gently ripple in the pond. Taking slow walks through the nearby forestry of a preserve. When we can, trips to the beach to relax in the sand or back home to visit family. These are the moments I cling to.

I've found that when you start measuring your life in months instead of years, you learn how to truly live. You stop making plans for "someday" and start doing the things that matter today. And that mindset, ironically, has made me more alive than I ever was before.

So yes, I'm dying. But more importantly—I'm living. Fiercely. Honestly. And with more love than I ever thought possible.

This isn't the end of my story. Not yet. It's just the beginning of a new way of living it.

CHAPTER 2: Where It All Began

I grew up in Milwaukee, Wisconsin, but my father was from Park Falls—a small paper mill town in northern Wisconsin, about five hours northwest of the Cream City. Park Falls was the kind of place where everyone knew everyone, where last names carried weight and history. For the Saunders family, that name was hard to miss. The city's largest source of revenue came from the paper mill, and the lumberyard that fed it bore our name. There was even a street named after my great-grandfather—Saunders Avenue. Original, I know.

Some of my earliest memories of my father's stories about Park Falls came at our kitchen table on the northwest side of Milwaukee. The table was scarred from decades of family meals and homework sessions, and it always smelled faintly of coffee. My dad would sit with his elbows resting on the surface, talking about growing up in a town where people didn't leave—not because they couldn't, but because they didn't want to. He married his high school sweetheart there, started a family young, and for a while, life followed the path it was supposed to.

That path didn't last.

For reasons that were never fully explained to me, my father's first marriage fell apart. Eventually, he decided to start over—finishing college, earning his Certified Public Accountant license, and moving to Milwaukee to begin a new chapter. His ex-wife and two children followed shortly after, keeping the family geographically close, at least on paper. At the time, that proximity seemed practical. In hindsight, it was the quiet beginning of a fracture that would widen over the years.

With a college degree and CPA license, he began his career in numbers, making stops at a handful of different companies. During one of these placements, my dad met a woman (my mother), and they began a relationship—a connection that would eventually blossom into a marriage and new family. It was a fresh start for my father and a chance to have the *normal* American family that he had once dreamed of in Park Falls.

My mother, on the other hand, has only known the city limits of Milwaukee. I picture her early life whenever I drive past the northeast side—brick houses pressed close together, church steeples rising above everything else. She spent most of her childhood on that side of Milwaukee and attended parochial schools from elementary through high school. Raised as a strict Roman Catholic, her large family of ten grew up in a very modest household, held together mostly by faith and religion.

My mom never went to college but instead entered the working world right out of high school. Various employments kept her busy and, as mentioned before, brought her to that fateful job where she met my father. After a whirlwind courtship, they were married in 1969 and quickly planted their roots on the northwest side of Milwaukee, an area that they would never leave.

I mention the Catholic upbringing because, growing up,

my mother was that bastion of Christianity that taught all of us what it meant to believe. We attended church every Sunday, in addition to attending during the week in school, and looked to my mother as our spiritual guide. I picture us sitting shoulder to shoulder in the wooden pews, knees pressed into the kneeler as we stood and sat on cue, my mother never missing a response. The rhythm of Mass was automatic—muscle memory as much as faith. She was strong in her convictions and eventually convinced my father to convert to Catholicism from Lutheranism. I never really thought of what it would have been like to grow up without religion in my life, rather it was just something that I understood to be inherently a part of my upbringing. And although I would not consider myself to be a very religious person today, I still believe in God and pray nightly, something that I've been thankful for throughout my life's challenges.

My parents quickly started a family of their own, bringing four children into this world between 1970 and 1975. Adam (*not his real name*) is four years my elder, Kelly is two, and Andrew is one year younger. After a brief stay in an apartment following Adam's birth, my parents purchased their first home together, a residence that my mom still occupies today (Note: this book has been many years in the making, and unfortunately, my father passed away in December of 2022). The other three of us were born in that home, and we all grew up in one consistent place, never leaving until we eventually went away to college.

Now, I say that I have three siblings, but more accurately, I also have a half-brother and half-sister from my dad's first marriage. My memories of seeing them as a child are kind of fuzzy, and I don't really recall how often that happened. There are photographs from those years that prove we spent time together—holiday snapshots, birthday cakes, forced smiles. I don't remember the moments themselves, only the spaces around them. I have zero recollection of ever meeting, or even seeing, my dad's ex-wife, but I seem to remember her being at their house when we'd go there, however she would "hide" in the other room from the rest of us. None of that seemed odd to me when I was young, and eventually the visits became less frequent and ultimately stopped. I'm sure my father would see his eldest children more often, but we certainly weren't a part of those later visits. As an adult, I came to find out that it was my mother, the "shining example of Christianity," that was the underlying reason for the eventual dissolution of our relationship with my half-siblings.

She was not fond of the fact that my father had been married before, and certainly not of the fact that he had other children. In the Catholic church, divorce was a dirty word, and she was embarrassed by the situation, actively doing what she could to hide it all behind a curtain. To think that she would go to the extremes that she did to paint this picture-perfect portrait of our lives, yet leaving out a huge portion of my father's life, really led me to question my faith later in life. How could someone, who preached the values of being a good Christian, ever treat anyone that way—her husband and his small children—it really made me wonder how much of what I had learned in school and at church was true. I didn't know it at the time, but the way my mom had handled this situation would be repeated over and over throughout our lives.

As I mentioned, my father held a handful of jobs as a CPA, but he always had a burning desire to own his own business. It was ingrained in him. His father owned multiple businesses, and both of his siblings went into business for themselves, so the yearning to be his own boss was something that he always carried with him.

He started small. He used the old motorhome that he had purchased years earlier to take our family on vacations when we were younger. Now that we had outgrown the traditional family road trip, he listed the tenement on wheels as a rental. It was mildly successful, but more than anything, it stoked the flames of wanting to build his own business. Eventually, he would expand that enterprise, adding more motorhomes to his "fleet" and the business started to grow. It was a constant source of busy work for my parents and occasionally pulled us kids in a bit, but it was also something that my parents could do together. Stressful from time to time, for sure, but it provided a sense of self-worth for both my father and mother. Ultimately, the small successes of this venture fed my dad's appetite for something more. He still wanted to live out that dream of owning his own business, and he was very determined to make it happen.

I was in high school when my father took the ultimate leap of faith. The motorhome business was something he could do on the side, but it hadn't released him from the corporate world that he had worked in for so many years. To capitalize on the success he was seeing with the rental business, he identified and purchased a gas station and repair shop, just a few miles from our home.

I remember the first time my dad took us there—the smell of oil and rubber hit before we even opened the car doors. The place felt smaller than I expected, cramped and loud, but he stood there smiling like he'd just claimed something enormous. He was now the owner and boss of his very own establishment.

It was mildly surprising, as he didn't have any experience in this industry, nor do I remember him being very hands-on with our own vehicles at home, but he was excited. We all were. For my parents, it was another chance to build a successful venture to support the family. For Adam and me, it eliminated the need to search for a part-time job during our teenage years. We had an opportunity to join the family business. That, of course, had its own set of pros and cons. We had steady work for as long as we'd like, but we were also always the fallback if someone didn't show up for work or got fired. If there was any shift that needed to be filled, we were always the first line of defense. I didn't mind as much, as I was younger and not quite as social as my brother, but we both did our share to help as often as we could. And the money was good—at least I think so. The hourly rate seemed higher than the other part-time jobs I had previously held, and my dad would pay me overtime in summer if I went over 40 hours a week.

Everything seemed to be going smoothly, at least as far as I could tell. My dad poured his heart and soul, and a lot of family finances, into making that business a success. What I didn't see, or at least was too young to understand, was what a strain on my parent's marriage that the gas station had become. My father put in a lot of hours and the family dynamic at home suffered. My dad wanted the business to succeed so badly, that he was willing to sacrifice whatever needed to be done to make that happen. Ultimately, what he sacrificed was a happy home.

My mother eventually stopped trying to hide her displeasure and our home on 100th Street became an uncomfortable place to be. She stopped masking her frustration. It showed up in sighs, clipped responses, and the way she stayed seated while my dad moved through the house. Evenings ended earlier. Lights went off in different rooms, doors closed without goodnights, and the house felt larger than it used to. The pressure for my dad to achieve what had seemingly come so easily to his siblings was more than he had anticipated but it didn't dampen his spirits or drive to succeed. Life pushed forward, but our family was never the same.

I worked at that gas station for most of my high school years, as well as the first summer after my freshman year of college, and although that place was a noted cause of anguish for our family, it wasn't always bad. My dad and I were fairly close growing up, but our time spent together at the station was probably the closest we had ever been or had been following. Not all my memories there were positive, but as this story continues, you'll see how it brought one of the greatest parts of my life to me.

I say that my dad and I were close growing up and that is certainly true. Looking back on it now, I may have been the child with the tightest relationship to my father. I wouldn't know it at the time, but I suspect that the bond was a little stronger because, in some ways, I'm a lot like him. Physical features, mannerisms and even his poor posture. Christina likes to mention it to me from time to time, how much I remind her of my dad, and I wear it as a badge of honor. My father was a great man, and I'm blessed to call him Dad.

In my younger years, I loved it. He was an assistant coach on my grade school basketball team and spent many hours at Cub Scout activities with me. For a time, he and I would run together after he got home from work and prior to dinner. We didn't always talk a lot on those runs, but it meant the world to me that we were running together. Honestly, it's probably the only reason I ran track in high school, and with those years of training, I was pretty good.

He was a solid football player in his day, so naturally he tried to push me into the game—signing me up for youth leagues and ultimately encouraging me to play in high school. Here's the problem, unlike my dad, I didn't hit my growth spurt until the summer between my Sophomore and Junior years. I "played" the first two years but was able to convince him to let me quit before Varsity. I mean, let's be honest here; I never played! I was a glorified tackling dummy in practice. And even that growth spurt, where I grew from 5'9" to 6'3" in the three months of summer, wasn't enough to keep me on the team. All that height, but only 135 lbs. isn't quite the physical presence the team was looking for. Still, I'm grateful for all that he did for me—even when I didn't agree with him. I love my father and miss him every day.

My relationship with my mother was good as well. We didn't have the "outside the home" activities that I shared with my father, but my mom's passion lied in the kitchen and none of us were upset about that. She is an amazing baker, which is something we all enjoyed. I also give her a lot of credit for her creativity when it came to dinner. The budget was tight, so it wasn't uncommon to have a meal, only to have that same meal in a different form the next night. She was a bit of a magician. I will also say that she is a very generous person by nature, almost to a fault. She will give you everything she has, without hesitation. She was there for me and Christina early in our marriage when we needed, but couldn't afford, childcare. We didn't take that for granted and were very appreciative. As this story goes on, you'll see how this generosity became a negative quality, but as I was growing up, she was all you could ask from a loving mother.

As a family, we did a lot of the *normal* family things. Early in life, when my dad worked as an accountant for a travel group, we had the chance to take some trips down to Florida to enjoy the weather and occasionally a theme park. Who knows, maybe that's where my desire to be a Florida resident someday came from. I was pretty young, so most of my memories from those trips are due to photographs, including having to navigate around Disney World with a cast that went all the way up my leg and around my waist. I had broken my leg shortly before at a family friend's BBQ and the timing was terrible. I know the bulk of the extra work fell squarely on my parents.

As time went on, trips with the full crew became less, and once my dad acquired that motorhome, it seemed like it was just him with Adam, Kelly and me. Occasionally we'd meet up with other relatives from other states, but the core was the four of us. My mom didn't like to travel. She hated flying and long drives were not her thing, so she and Andrew would stay back at home. Andrew was also a bit of a wildcard (more on that later), so rather than open us up to potential situations on the road, they stayed back.

Outside of those trips, a lot of the memories I have revolve around family gatherings. With such a large family on my mom's side, there always seemed to be a reason to celebrate or just get together. In town, we saw each other a lot. My dad's side of the family in Northern Wisconsin, however, we didn't get to see quite as much. It was a commitment to go that far, but when we did, we had the time of our lives. So many cousins and so much mischief to get into. Houses by lakes, boats, tubes, waterskiing. It was a blast.

Life in my younger years felt *normal*.

INTERLUDE: Rumple What?

I never played high school basketball. By the time I had the height, it was too late. I had that growth spurt between my sophomore and junior year and was suddenly grabbing rebounds like it was nothing—but I'd already missed my window. I remember playing intramural hoops one afternoon when the school's basketball coach stopped me mid-game and asked, *"How come you never tried out for the basketball team?"*

I shot back, *"How come you never knew who I was before?"*

He nodded. *"That's fair."*

By then, though, I wasn't interested in tryouts or running suicides. I was more interested in partying and living it up. Still, I found a loophole—the Christian Youth Organization (CYO) team. A few of my buddies played, and we took it just seriously enough to show up. Most games consisted of sneaking a few beers beforehand, playing terribly, and then celebrating afterward like we'd just won March Madness.

On one particular night following a game, I was introduced to the icy regret that is Rumple Minze. I was 15. I had never tasted that minty menace before, and I definitely didn't know how potent it was. After taking down a healthy portion of the bottle, I figured it was time to call it a night and walk the block and a half home. It was late—or at least it felt late—and I was sure my parents would be asleep.

I was wrong.

I stumbled through the door and there they were—my parents, sitting at the kitchen table, looking at me like I had walked in on fire. I mumbled something about not feeling well and headed straight for the downstairs bathroom. They followed. I tried to shut the door and ride it out alone, but my mom wasn't having it. She knocked, then demanded I open up. The moment she stepped in, she knew.

I was a drunk 15-year-old mess, clinging to the edge of the toilet.

They sat me on the couch, and my mom held the barf bucket in between calls to the detox center, trying to figure out if this was hospital-worthy. It was overkill, maybe—but she was terrified.

And then, just to complete the picture, my brother Adam stumbled in, equally hammered—he was 19, so also not drunk legally. He took one look at the scene, burst out laughing, and yelled, *"Ohhhh, Matt's drunk!"* before my dad redirected him to bed like a misbehaving toddler.

In the moment, I was mortified. I thought my life was over.

But a couple weeks later, I was riding in the car with my dad when we passed a billboard for Rumple Minze. He just pointed and chuckled. That's when I knew—despite everything—his small-town roots and big-picture perspective had kicked in. He found the humor in it. Eventually, so did I.

I've never touched Rumple Minze since. Some lessons you only need to learn once.

CHAPTER 3: A Normal Childhood…Sort Of

Milwaukee, Wisconsin is not a big city. Sure, the people that call Milwaukee home would like to think it's a big city, but to be perfectly honest, it's a large "small town." It's not without some notable attractions, however. This "Great Place by a Great Lake" is home to the 2021 NBA Champion Milwaukee Bucks, the Milwaukee Brewers have been around since 1970, Miller Brewing and Harley Davidson were born and raised in the Cream City and Summerfest, once the world's largest music festival held annually every summer, is nestled along a one-mile stretch of Lake Michigan. I'd be lying if I said we didn't look an hour to the south at Chicago and all that city has to offer with some degree of jealousy, but Milwaukee has quite a bit to offer (ahem—without all the traffic) and is a great place to live. I'd argue that the winters might negate anything worth experiencing in this city, but overall, it's worth a summertime visit if you've never had the pleasure of passing through this blue-collar town.

I grew up in a modest 3-bedroom house on the northwest side of Milwaukee, eventually sharing one small room with my two brothers, so my sister could have her own space. When you're a kid, you don't really mind sharing, but years later, when my dad had the basement finished to include two additional bedrooms and a second bathroom, the extra space was welcomed, for sure. Six people squeezed into a small house seems awful now, but at the time, I loved every minute of it. The closer we were to each other physically, the more we bonded as a family.

The community was nice, our neighbors were friendly, and although there seemed be an inordinate number of older couples living near us, there were plenty of kids and friends our age in the vicinity as well. Summers were spent on bikes or skateboards, annoying those older neighbors. Cell phones didn't exist, so we'd say goodbye to our moms in the morning, hop on our bikes to explore the day, not returning home until dinner was on the table. We filled our time doing nothing in particular, but somehow it was exactly what we wanted to do.

When I wasn't out burning the trails on my bike, I'd use the free time to make a little spending cash. My brother had a paper route that I would help with from time to time, but for the most part, I found the easy money was in lawn mowing and snow shoveling. One of the perks of having aging neighbors is that they were more than willing to pass off the lawncare and snow removal responsibilities to a kid for a nominal cost. To me, every little bit seemed like a lot, so sweating it out behind a mower or chillingly pushing a shovel, was worth the $10-$15 reward.

In all honesty, most of these "customers" were looking as much for someone to talk to as they were about having their lawn curated or sidewalk cleared. I remember one neighbor who had just lost his wife, and visits to cut his lawn usually included a long conversation afterwards. On one occasion, I was invited in for a glass of lemonade to cool down after sweating through the job. I accepted and took a seat in the lounge chair in his living room. As he approached with my drink, he dropped the unfiltered anecdote that I was sitting in his wife's favorite chair. I was understandably uncomfortable, but it escalated quickly when he said, *"Yep, that's the chair Theresa died in. One cough and she let out her last breath."* I couldn't get out of that chair fast enough. I jumped up and told him I forgot that I had another lawn job I needed to attend to. I grabbed my cash, set down my drink and hastily headed for the door. When I got home and told my parents, they couldn't stop laughing. For years, that story was shared like an urban legend, only I knew there was nothing legendary about it.

My specific neighborhood was one of those communities where friendships and acquaintances were abundant. In particular, the families that sent their children to St. Margaret Mary grade school and attended weekly mass at STMM certainly all knew each other. Trips to the store were never quick, as our parents would inevitably run into at least one other STMM family, and the conversation would seemingly go on forever. Being treated to dinner at a restaurant always seemed to include a family or two that we knew at tables nearby. And as a kid, the 15-20 block radius surrounding our house seemed like the entire world. Anything outside of that perimeter was almost like a completely different planet.

Your friends were your classmates and, since my school was 5K-8th grade, we spent just about our entire adolescent lives together. After school, we spilled onto the sidewalks in clusters, backpacks bouncing as we fanned out toward our houses. By dinner, we'd circle back again. As a kid, you grow up thinking these will be the only people in your life forever. You went to school together, went to church together, played sports together and filled every waking moment in the summers together. First girlfriends, school dances, Cub scouts and Friday fish fries—we felt like, outside of the 5-mile radius around STMM, nothing else existed, and we definitely weren't thinking about life after grade school.

One of my fondest memories from the STMM days, was also an ironic precursor to the connections life can make. My final year in elementary school was dominated by an overzealous teacher who loved the theater and was determined to pull off a stage performance of *The Wizard of Oz*. I'm sure my mind is exaggerating this memory, but it seemed like we spent that entire school year in the gymnasium basement, auditioning, building backdrops, rehearsing and ultimately performing the play. It was a combined effort between the 7th and 8th grade classes, and it was a blast.

I don't truly know where the courage came from (I must have channeled my "inner Lion"), but I auditioned for and got the part of the Tin Man. I dove headfirst into that role and diligently memorized all my lines. What I didn't know at first, but eventually powered through, was that this role, amongst others, included a solo singing performance. There I was, with my squeaky voice, belting out what was likely a horrible rendition of *If I Only Had a Heart*.

Little did I know, staring at me from the row of Poppies in front of the stage, occasionally singing along to the tunes of the musical, was my future wife. We still laugh about it from time to time and if we ever want to be transported back to that gym basement, my father-in-law still has a VHS copy of the performance. Small world indeed, but it serves as an example of the even smaller community we grew up in.

As I got older, the picture of the real world started to come into focus. The first morning I arrived at Marquette University High School, I stepped out onto Wisconsin Avenue and felt like I'd landed somewhere entirely different. The buildings were bigger, the streets louder, and the edges of the neighborhood sharper than anything I'd known.

Until then, I hadn't realized that our happy little existence in near-suburban Milwaukee wasn't the norm across the city. Milwaukee has long been one of the most segregated cities in America, and it took me years to fully understand what that meant. High school was where my eyes first opened. MUHS, one of the most respected schools in the state, sat on the edge of downtown, at 35th and Wisconsin Avenue—an all-boys, college-prep school surrounded by a neighborhood that looked nothing like the one most of my classmates went home to at the end of the day.

What MUHS really did was open my eyes to how much I didn't yet understand about the world—and about myself. My parents worked hard to afford sending me there, and while I didn't grow up with much, I had more than I realized at the time. Still, the new landscape felt isolating.

The halls felt louder than they needed to be—lockers slamming, voices bouncing off cinderblock walls—while I moved through it all like background noise. I stuck to the edges, backpack tight to my shoulder, counting minutes until the bell rang.

I worked hard to afford my first car, and I was proud of my accomplishment, but every morning of my Junior and Senior years, when I pulled into the parking lot in my 1974 Volkswagen Beetle, that car looked wildly out of place next to the Mercedes-Benzes and BMWs my classmates drove. At first, that contrast made me feel smaller. But over time, it taught me something important. I may have had less than most of the students at MUHS, but I had far more than many people just a few blocks away who were struggling to survive.

Those four years changed the way I saw opportunity. I stopped assuming things would be handed to me and started learning how to earn what came next. I didn't fully understand it then, but that mindset—work hard, stay humble, seize what's in front of you—was taking root.

As far as my family dynamic, I could not have been happier. I'm sure there were minor sibling disputes that I've erased from my memory, but for the most part, we were a tight knit group. When my dad worked for that travel corporation, we were lucky enough to take those trips down to Florida to meet Mickey Mouse. As time went on, those flights changed to those motorhome rides to visit landmarks around the United States. Life was great. I had a good relationship with my parents despite a few incidents that really tested their patience, and overall, we were a loving family that truly cared for each other. Everything seemed *normal*.

My extended family on my mom's side was also nearby, and we got together with them often. Walking home from school frequently involved a stop along the way to say *"hi"* to my grandmother and inspect her kitchen for baked goods. A couple of my aunts and one of my cousins lived there as well, so a short stop definitely turned into an extended visit. My cousin was two years older than me and was exactly two days older than my sister, so it really felt like he was just another sibling, rather than a cousin. Family gatherings and holidays formally brought us all together, but honestly, we were always by each other's sides without any of those occasions.

When my grandmother unexpectedly passed away during my eighth-grade school year, everything felt different. After the funeral, we gathered at her house like we always had—but something was off. People stood in corners instead of sitting down, conversations lowering whenever someone new entered the room. She was the glue that held the extended family together and the ugliness that ensued after her passing was not pleasant. Arguments over her house and keepsakes were one thing, but it was nothing compared to the spitefulness that arose when it came to the little bit of money she left behind. Honestly, my world was different after that. The visits slowed almost immediately. What had once been automatic—stopping by, lingering, laughing—now required planning, and often didn't happen at all. I didn't know it at the time, but the way the adults were treating each other during a trying time that should have brought everyone closer together, was a precursor to issues we would experience in our immediate family in the future.

Luckily for me, the youngsters in the family didn't let the pettiness of the adults get in our way. Like I said, we were a tight knit group and none of that changed after my grandmother's passing. We all went to different schools, but evenings and weekends would always bring us together to hang out, go to the movies or do whatever seemed right. It was a time of discovery, for sure, and what I didn't know, being one of the youngest of the group, was how much discovery was actually going on.

Adam and my cousin, Jason (not his real name), were very close and spent a lot of time together. My sister, being the same age as Jason, also spent a lot of time with the group, but luckily, she was a very intelligent and level-headed girl that knew her limits. Adam and Jason, on the other hand, tested the boundaries as often as they could. I'm not completely sure what all went on back in those days, but I know that sneaking some drinks, like any *normal* teenager, was just the tip of the iceberg for those two and their friends. Unconfirmed stories of parties with various substances have been rehashed over the years, but I never really knew what to believe. We all know kids like to exaggerate stories to build up some "street credibility" but knowing what I know now, and the trajectory that Adam's life in particular took, I must believe that there was a lot of truth to those stories.

As I got older and was able to be a more permanent part of the circle, I'm not sure if things had calmed down a bit or if they purposely kept some of those shenanigans away from me, but I never saw the craziness that had been passed along from story to story.

I tell these stories, not to make myself out to be this perfect child. Unfortunately, I was far from it, and as mentioned earlier, I tested my parent's patience from time to time. I mean, the PG-rated tales really revolve around stupid things like getting caught underage drinking at a remote lake 30-minutes from home. Not a big deal, as far as I was concerned, but the end of the world to someone like my mom. She grew up in a family of alcoholics, and she unfortunately watched a couple of her siblings drink themselves into an early grave. So, having to pick her 16-year-old son up from the small-town police station and weeks later drive him to court to get reamed out by the judge, meant a little more to her than just being disappointed in my poor judgement.

Not much phased me, unfortunately, and I continued to test the limits. One particular evening, a group of friends and I decided, after a few "cold ones", that it would be a good idea to take some target practice with a BB gun. As the evening progressed and our friend who hadn't had anything to drink offered to drive us around, we decided it would be fun to expand the marks to street signs and moving targets. Never one to think too far ahead at potential consequences, I decided it would be fun to see if a BB would bounce off a car tire and what would come next. We sat at a stoplight, and I took aim at the tire of the car waiting next to us. As I lined up the shot and got ready to pull the trigger, one of my friends thought it would be funny to shove me, throwing my aim way off. The BB gun went off, hitting the passenger side window of the occupied vehicle, shattering the glass into an infinite number of pieces.

We panicked. Our driver hit the gas and quickly maneuvered into a nearby neighborhood. The car with the broken window followed close behind, trying to get the license plate number. Eventually, I asked my friend to stop the car so we could get out and make sure everyone in the other vehicle was okay. As we came to a stop, so did the other car, waiting just long enough to grab our plate number and speed away.

I think I knew at that point that this was bigger than any other stupid stunt I had pulled before. The four of us in the car decided to do what every other teenager in that situation would do—lie. We came up with a story about how we were sitting at the light and saw a car window shatter, so we panicked and sped off so we wouldn't get hit by whatever caused the damage. We eventually stopped to check on the other car, but they left the scene. It seemed logical and like a good story, one that we all told our parents when we got home. As suspected, the police made their way to the home of the friend who was driving. He held strong and told our tale to the cops. They subsequently visited all our homes over the next couple of hours, hearing the same story from each of us. I went to bed thinking that we had pulled one over and were in the clear.

At about 2 am, my father stood at the threshold of my bedroom, and he somberly instructed me to get up and get dressed. I asked what was going on, but he simply turned his back and walked away with a very solemn look on his face. I got dressed and walked to the living room to find the same police officers who had questioned me earlier in the night. They walked up, looked me square in the eyes and asked me to repeat my story, only this time, they wanted the truth. Apparently, their final stop, at one of my friend's houses, was too much for him and his parents. He cracked and told the police everything, including where to find the BB gun.

I was stuck. Nowhere to run but to the truth. So, I revised my story, told them what had actually happened, but explained that it was an accident. None of it resonated, and they had a job to do so they stood up, asked me to turn around and announced that they were placing me under arrest. Handcuffs were slapped on my wrists, and I was walked out to the police car waiting out front. I remember thinking how I was glad that it was 2am, so not many, if any, of the neighbors would be watching my walk of shame. I never did find out if anyone saw, but I'd have to assume some of those nosy neighbors caught a glimpse.

The handcuffs were one thing and the walk to the police car was another, but the real punch in the gut was having to walk by my parents, head down and being escorted by a cop, as my mother stood there, sobbing. It was quite possibly the worst feeling I had ever had to that point in my life, and I don't think I've ever felt that embarrassed or disappointed in myself since. At the age of 16, I had experienced what felt like the lowest of the low. I felt awful for putting my parents through this, but it was only the beginning.

I was taken to a local Milwaukee precinct to continue being questioned. Still in handcuffs, still trying to understand how something so stupid had spiraled so fast, I sat there waiting while officers decided what to do with me next. One of my cousins—who was a Milwaukee police officer at the time—stepped in and made sure I wasn't placed in a holding cell with the other detainees. Instead, I was kept alone in an interrogation room for the next few hours while everything was sorted out.

I didn't yet understand how serious this was. I knew I was in trouble, but I was still clinging to the idea that it would end with a lecture, maybe a call home, something manageable. I had no real sense of what was coming.

That clarity didn't arrive until the next day, when I was driven downtown to the main precinct.

That's where I was fully processed. Fingerprints. Mug shots. Paperwork. And that's where I finally heard the charge read out loud: reckless endangerment with a deadly weapon. I was floored. What had started as a thoughtless stunt—one with no intention of harming anyone—had now become a serious criminal charge, one that could land me in adult court. Hearing those words made everything feel suddenly permanent.

After it was over, I was driven home. Free to leave, but shaken by how close I had come to a very different outcome.

It was all a whirlwind, and with a charge that included the words "deadly weapon," I was convinced this was it for me. I honestly believed I'd spend at least the rest of my teenage years in jail somewhere. This is where my high school—and, to be very honest, my white privilege—took the wheel.

My parents, desperate to help me out any way they could, were able to connect with a lawyer whose son had been a student at MUHS. He was a prominent lawyer in Milwaukee, one that would two years later represent and defend notorious serial killer, Jeffrey Dahmer, in his high-profile case. He would certainly come at a high price tag as well. All things that you take for granted as a young and foolish kid, but at the time were relieved to find out.

I returned home the following day, and after a little pep talk from the officer who drove me back to my parents, they welcomed me with huge hugs. The officer explained what a trying ordeal I had gone through, especially once I arrived downtown to the taunts and jeers of the much older inmates, and he cautioned that they should go easy on me. I truly appreciate, not only what that officer did, but for the response that my parents gave me. They understood that I had already been punished in a way, and that yelling at me or grounding me at this point was likely going to pale in comparison.

Not much time passed before I went for my first appearance before the judge. I met with my lawyer and he let me know how the day would go. After leaving the room for a bit, he returned to inform us that he had worked out some details with the judge, outside of the courtroom, and if I pled no contest, I would only be subject to a year of probation. Any slip ups in the next 12 months and I most certainly would have had to face the judge, but the events of the last few weeks were enough to scare me straight.

Looking back on it now, the incident was an eye-opener and,

although I'd make some questionable decisions in the years to come, nothing would compare to the level of severity of this one. I also think of the events of that day in court and how, had I not been a white male, attending a prestigious high school that afforded me some enhanced resources, would I have walked away with a slap on the wrist like I did? I truly believe the answer to that question is a resounding "no" and has been a source of my empathy for the damaged society that we live in. All I could do, and strive to do every day, is understand those societal differences and do whatever I can in my power to make the world a better place for all.

INTERLUDE: A Taste of Victory

Milwaukee may be a small market, but when it comes to its sports teams, the residents of Cream City have huge hearts. In 1987, just a few years after the Brewers had reached the pinnacle of the sport—only to fall short in the World Series to the St. Louis Cardinals—they started the season on fire. Thirteen straight wins to open the year. It was electric. I mean, I was already a baseball fan, but this run really solidified the love affair I still have with the Brew Crew (sometimes, painstakingly). Sure, they would go on to lose twelve in a row the very next month, but in April, the entire city had Brewer fever.

There's a small restaurant chain in Milwaukee called George Webb's. It's a classic greasy spoon that serves exactly what you'd expect—eggs and bacon in the morning (although you could get breakfast all day) and double cheeseburgers all night. The originator of George Webb's was also a big Brewers fan, and for as far back as I can remember, they had a standing promise: if the Brew Crew ever won twelve games in a row, they'd give away free hamburgers to the entire city.

When that 12th win hit, it was chaos—in the best way. It's hard to say whether people were more excited about the

Brewers' success or the free food, but the lines on the day George Webb's fulfilled its promise were miles long. We stood in line at three different locations that day, loading up on as many burgers as we could. Not because they were anything special, but because they were free. And because they symbolized something remarkable in Milwaukee's sports history.

Those burgers were mass-produced, lukewarm, and probably not the tastiest things we ever ate. But they sure tasted like victory.

CHAPTER 4: Life's First Blessing

When I think back to my childhood, I try to pinpoint the moment I realized my brother Andrew was different. We were almost exactly a year apart, so I was still young during his early hospital stays. Visiting him at St. Joseph's became *normal*—holding my mother's hand as we walked down long, echoing hallways that smelled like antiseptic. When it was time to leave, I didn't understand why he stayed behind. I distinctly recall the summer of 1979, right around my 5th and Andrew's 4th birthdays. My parents let me know that Andrew was "coming home for good" and I was so excited. I remember standing in our front doorway, watching my parents bring Andrew inside, not realizing that something permanent had just changed. To me, it just felt like the best surprise I'd ever gotten.

Andrew and I grew up reaching milestones at about the same time and I never really thought he was different, but eventually, when Andrew didn't join us at STMM, I began to question why. He went to St. Coletta's Day School in a different part of town, so you can imagine my confusion when he was venturing off to school completely separate of his three siblings. Eventually, when I was old enough to understand, my parents sat me down at the kitchen table, the same one where we ate dinner every night. They spoke carefully, slowly, as if the words themselves might break something, eventually explaining that Andrew had been born with Down syndrome. They emphasized that while he looked and spoke a little differently, he was still my brother—and deserved to be treated just like Adam or Kelly. It had to be a difficult conversation for my parents, as I was pretty young and likely didn't understand completely, but the one thing I didn't need them to tell me was to treat Andrew the same way as everyone else. He's my brother—of course I'm going to love him just like Adam and Kelly. As the years went on, however, I began to understand why they felt the need to tell me that. The world can be a cruel place and anyone that's labeled as "different" certainly has it tougher than most. I watched in anger as people would stare at my brother and I definitely got in my fair share of altercations, defending Andrew from anyone who would verbally abuse him.

Technically, Down syndrome is caused by an extra copy of chromosome 21, which affects development—but calling it a "condition" never sat right with me. The word feels cold and clinical. Andrew is not a condition. He's a person—and one of the best people I know. The negative connotation that comes along with "having a condition" is, in my opinion, the primary factor behind why people don't understand and ultimately treat individuals with Down syndrome differently. Now, the heart disease that Andrew had to endure early in his life, that is certainly a condition, but I will not accept being born with Down syndrome as a condition.

If you haven't had the pleasure of interacting with a child or adult with Down syndrome, I have to say that you're missing out. They are the most loving and honest human beings on the face of the earth. Andrew is no exception, and he wears his heart on his sleeve for just about everything—family, sports teams, food, and soap operas. If he had to give any of those up, I'm not sure how he'd survive. I feel truly blessed to have had Andrew in my life for 50 years and I can say unequivocally that he has helped shape me into the man that I am today. The unconscious biases that plague all humans are more apparent to me, and I've spent a lifetime trying to ensure that I don't succumb to these preconceptions when encountering someone for the first time. It's not always easy but having Andrew in my life gave me the head start necessary to approach all people the same way—the right way.

As the years have gone on and for reasons I will discuss later, Andrew and I have lost touch with each other, and it absolutely kills me inside. It didn't happen all at once. Looking back, the distance crept in quietly, until one day I realized we were no longer part of each other's daily lives.

In addition to being brothers of just about the same age, Andrew has always been the source of the best stories in our lives. The little things he'd do to entertain the family are moments that I will always cherish—and miss the most.

Whether it was looking back after finally clearing all the snow from the sidewalk, only to find Andrew shoveling it back onto the cement, or his unannounced walks to the local grocery store where he'd use the credit card my parents reluctantly acquired for him to "pick up the check" from time to time (he loved that), to load up on ice cream that melted completely on his walk home, the memories are abundant.

I was a little jealous that I ended up being the last kid in the family to drive a car, but in his typical fashion, Andrew stole the show (and my dad's car for a minute) to get behind the wheel before either of us legally could. We were having a family gathering at my parent's house and it got hectic, as it always did. At some point in the afternoon, someone shouted out the frequently asked question back in the day, *"Where's Andrew?"* We didn't have to search long before discovering that he had grabbed my dad's car keys and locked himself in the front seat of the woody wagon. This was 1986, so I was 12 and Andrew was only 11, but he had no concept that he wasn't supposed to be doing this. He had watched my parents drive the car over the years and apparently picked up enough information to figure out how to do it by himself. So as the party rushed to the front yard to stop whatever he was about to do, Andrew had already had the car running and was about to put it in gear.

I mentioned the woody wagon because, for anyone old enough to remember, those classics had the seat in the rear that faced backwards (safe, I know—I don't even think there were seatbelts back there) and a power sliding glass window that you could open via a switch near the driver. Prior to assuming his spot as the captain on that day, Andrew typically would get in the car with my family and the first thing he'd do was reach for the switch to roll that back window down. On this day, it was a blessing that he had done just that because as he put the car in gear, turned sharply to the left and drove up my neighbor's lawn, put it in reverse and brought the car back on the street, for a brief moment in time, he stopped and that was my chance to spring to action. With the car not moving, I jumped through the back window and quickly climbed through the car towards the front. As I got near Andrew, who was laughing hysterically, he decided it was time to slam on the brakes. The short gap closed in an instant as

I was hurled into the front seat. I grabbed the gear shift and put the car in park. Andrew had just pulled off the world's largest Y-turn, one that included some very large ruts in the neighbor's lawn. I unlocked the doors, and my parents opened the front door to grab Andrew and make sure both of us were okay. When the dust had settled, we laughed and laughed as we rehashed the story all night, and for years to come.

It's worth mentioning, as an example of the good neighbors we had around us, that the family across the street refused to let my dad pay to have their lawn fixed. They, like everyone that has met him, loved Andrew and declined any attempts my dad made for financial retribution. I don't remember those neighbor's names, but they are a shining example of someone that appreciated the joy that Andrew brought, and still brings, to everyone's life. He's a special person and I miss him dearly.

As the years went on and Adam, Kelly and I navigated through the next steps of our lives, the gap between our milestones and Andrew's was widening. Sure, he was involved in sports through Special Olympics, and he had a part-time job at the local grocery store, but our paths were shaping up much differently. Andrew would eventually enjoy the satisfaction of graduating from high school, but college wasn't in his future. He likely would have thrived in an assisted living facility with friends that shared the same cognitive disabilities, but my mother felt it best to keep him at home. I was sad for Andrew, thinking about "what could have been" but if you asked him, he wouldn't want his life to change a bit.

Andrew lived for those Special Olympics events, and much like his siblings, he had a flair for entertainment. Watching what the pros do and how they celebrate every moment may not have been the best thing for Andrew, as he emulated all those celebrations every chance he got. I recall one bocce ball tournament, where Andrew had a safe lead, so he decided to throw his next ball between his legs—something he had already been warned not to do. Disqualified, yes, but if I said we didn't laugh about that moment for years afterwards, I'd be lying. And you never would have known the eventual victory had been stripped from him due to his antics. Andrew wore it as a badge of honor.

Working as a bagger at the local grocery store (the same store where he purchased and subsequently melted that ice cream) might seem boring and mundane to some, but Andrew attacked that job with the same energy and enthusiasm that he did with everything in his life. Frequently offering to take the groceries out to the car and assist with loading, Andrew displayed a huge heart every chance he got. His biggest hurdle was having to decline the inevitable tips that people would offer him. Andrew is a very likable guy, and if you sprinkle in his kind heart and willingness to help, $2 here and $5 there was not uncommon. He's also an honest guy, so any time he received a tip, he took it to his manager, and the money was put into a fund for small employee outings or picnics. I have to think Andrew supplied most of the funding to support those events.

On one occasion, my mom picked Andrew up from work, with his snack and soda in hand (it was his routine—every shift), she asked, as she always did, *"How was work?"* Like clockwork, Andrew would reply *"Good."* Hours later, the phone rang, and my mom answered. It was Andrew's manager, checking to see how he was doing. My mother was understandably confused and asked why he was inquiring. To her surprise, the manager said the store had been robbed that day, and Andrew was very close to the "action." Apparently, it was quite the scene with a gun being brandished and some pushing and shoving before the suspect raced out of the store.

But Andrew, he didn't do anything and, in fact, froze in his tracks, and when the commotion was over, he simply went back to his job, thinking nothing of what had just transpired. Classic Andrew! We liked to joke over the years that Andrew, being a pretty big guy, probably just turned his body sideways, thinking that if he could make himself as thin as a piece of paper, the thief wouldn't see him.

I mentioned that we have drifted apart and will provide those difficult details shortly, but I'm proud to say that Andrew's legacy lives on in my household. My kids truly adore Uncle Andrew. If I thought he was funny, the kids find him exponentially hilarious. Andrew is the reason why my kids call me by my unofficial nickname. Growing up, Andrew followed the same path of most adolescents with Down syndrome, and he put on quite a few pounds over the years. Affectionately, and within the theme of 90's hip-hop, I called him Chunky A. I wouldn't say he loved that nickname, but he embraced it. Of course, he felt the need to assign me a moniker as well, and the first thing he thought of was to call me Mattress. I mean, of all the options out there, he came up with Mattress? Well, my children find that to be extremely comical, and to this day, they will periodically call me Mattress, but I'm okay with it because it reminds me of him.

Just a small sampling of the World of Andrew. Phrases that we still utter, all with an "Andrew accent":

"Yeah, white!" which is supposed to be *"Yeah, right!"*

"Whenever!" which apparently is meant to be *"Whatever!"*

And my personal favorite—when he couldn't remember

something, he'd combine "forget and remember" to be *"Uh, I formember."*

Honestly, I could fill a book with Andrew stories. He's real. He's honest. He's generous and loving in a way most people only aspire to be. The world might see Andrew as different, but in so many ways, he's the most *normal* person I've ever known.

CHAPTER 5: Sibling Love

I'd be remiss if I didn't mention my other two siblings, Adam and Kelly. The three of us grew up stacked on top of each other in a small house—too many people, not enough room, and nowhere to hide. You learned quickly how to coexist, or at least how to survive. Like I said before, I'm sure there have been moments when we were at each other's throats, but for the most part, my memories are all good ones. I recall looking up to Adam and Kelly and have always loved them unconditionally.

Adam had the pleasure, or depending on how you looked at it, the pressure, of being the first born. Adam was an adventurous kid who, as the years went on would test the family's patience, but in our younger years, he was just another *normal* kid, doing all those adolescent activities I talked about earlier. Adam, more than any of the other kids, loved the city of Milwaukee, vowing that he'd never leave. Now, he also said he wouldn't live to see the age of 40, but I'm getting ahead of myself. He has a zest for life that is at the same time, admirable and destructive. More on that in a bit.

Kelly has always been so good to me, even at a young age. While Adam was busy blazing his own trail—sometimes with gasoline and a match—Kelly was the quiet strength in our house. She was patient when the rest of us were chaos, kind when tempers flared, and wise beyond her years. If Adam was the storm and I was the curiosity-fueled tornado, Kelly was the calm that followed.

She had this uncanny ability to read a room before anyone else walked in. I don't know if it was intuition or just growing up in a crowded house with three brothers and parents constantly juggling stress, but she always knew what people needed—even if they didn't know it themselves. I remember once, after a particularly bad day at school when I had gotten into it with a teacher and came home ready to break something, Kelly didn't say a word. She just handed me one of her homemade chocolate chip cookies and sat next to me in silence. That moment probably did more for me than any lecture ever could.

Kelly didn't just mother us when things were tense—she celebrated us when things were good. Birthdays, report cards, small victories—she made everything feel like a moment worth marking. And when Andrew needed the extra love and attention that sometimes pulled focus, she never once complained. She loved him fiercely, and I think watching how she loved him taught me how to be a better brother—not just to Andrew, but to all my siblings.

Kelly has always been a teacher. Long before she ever stepped into a classroom with a lesson plan and a roster, she was already showing the rest of us how to learn—not just about books, but about life. She went on to become a wildly successful English teacher, shaping hundreds, maybe thousands, of young minds with the same mix of passion, patience, and empathy that she poured into our family. But long before she was Ms. Saunders to her students, she was just Kelly—my big sister, my academic safety net, and in many ways, my emotional compass.

She was the one who'd help me rewrite a paper the night before it was due—not because I asked, but because she could tell I needed help. She somehow made me feel smarter without making me feel small. It wasn't just about grammar and sentence structure, though heaven knows I needed the help—it was that she believed in me. Even when I didn't. Especially when I didn't.

Her support has never been limited to red pens and motivational speeches. She has shown up for me in every way imaginable. Financially, there were times in my life when I was down, and she stepped in without hesitation. She never made me feel ashamed, never treated her help like a loan that came with guilt attached. It was just what she did and continues to do. That's who she is. If she has it, you have it too. Simple as that.

Emotionally, she's been a quiet lifeline. She's always known when to reach out, when to give space, and when to just be there. No conditions, no expectations. Just presence. There are few things more grounding than knowing someone loves you without agenda, and that's the gift Kelly has always given me.

And then there's the inclusion—those unforgettable moments that might seem small from the outside but meant the world to me. Like when she was a student at the University of Wisconsin and took me, her still-in-high-school kid brother, to see Pearl Jam at a small bar in Madison. It was before they were huge—before they were playing arenas—and we were packed into this dive bar with a few hundred people, sweat dripping from the ceiling, the music vibrating through the floorboards. I remember thinking, this is what it feels like to matter. To be seen. To be let into a world I didn't think I belonged in yet. Kelly gave me that.

When Kelly made the move to the Pacific Northwest for grad school at the University of Washington, she made sure I was able to visit. Helping with airfare, giving me a place to stay and being the greatest tour guide of the city of Seattle. I still talk about those trips fondly and I attribute my zest for travel and exploration to Kelly. She has always preached about living life to the fullest and not getting wrapped up in little things that can hold you back. You only have a place on this earth once, so take advantage of all the opportunities while they are there.

I always saw Kelly as a studious, well-behaved, golden child in my youth, and I wouldn't say I was too far off, but there is another side of Kelly that I'm blessed to have discovered. She's taught me a lot. I just mentioned the travel, but I can attribute my love of film and music to her as well. We have always shared a similar ear when it came to music, and her living in the epicenter of the Grunge phase of the 1990's made those trips extra exciting. We'd sightsee based solely on music and films—Kurt Cobain and Courtney Love's house, Jimi Hendrix's grave, and the exterior shots filmed in Seattle of two of our favorite movies, *Say Anything* and *Singles*.

It shouldn't have come as a surprise to me when she told me during one of our phone calls, that a certain someone, from a band I loved, had been wooing her at the bars. I, of course, didn't believe her, but I listened to the stories while plotting my plan to expose her the next time I was in Seattle for a visit. When the time came and I was there for my next adventure, we were sitting at her apartment, nursing hangovers and deciding what to eat. The phone rang and it was her friend, offering us free tickets to see another favorite, Dinosaur Jr., at a small club. Headache be damned, I was all in. We quickly got ready, grabbed a cab and headed to the show.

Wouldn't you know it, the moment we walked in, the bandmember suitor she had told me about was there, along with the rest of the band (you may have heard of them—they call themselves Soundgarden). As one of the other bandmates walked near us, I nudged my sister and gave her a sarcastic, *"There's your buddies. Why don't you say hi?"* I barely got the words out of my mouth, just as he approached us, said "hello" to Kelly and gave her a huge hug. I just stood there with my jaw on the floor. My plan was foiled, but it was such a cool moment. And that's who Kelly is—she has a knack for being in those memorable occasions and she is always willing to bring me along for the ride.

Years later, as a high school English teacher, she started a film studies program at her school and somehow found a way to bring me along as a "chaperone" for their annual trip to the Sundance Film Festival. Let's be clear—I was there for the movies, not the minors. But that's Kelly. She creates these incredible experiences for others and then finds a way to bring the people she loves into them, too. Those trips were unforgettable—not just for the films or the mountain air, but because it was a front-row seat to watch my sister in her element: passionate, driven, and relentlessly inclusive.

She has always had that magic—to make people feel like they belong exactly where they are. She's done that for her students, her friends, her colleagues, and most importantly, she's done that for me. Through every diagnosis, every detour, every moment when I thought the weight of life might crush me, she has lifted me back up.

If there's one thread running through this entire story I'm telling, it's that family—real family—holds you up when everything else falls. And Kelly, for me, has been the scaffolding more times than I can count.

We likely had our differences like anyone (although I don't recall any specific examples), but I can say with absolute certainty that Kelly has always had my back. Even when I didn't deserve it. Especially when I didn't deserve it. Through the messiness of my teen years, all the way through the diagnoses I struggled to understand or explain away, she stayed close. She didn't excuse everything—but she never let me feel alone.

When I got sick—really sick—Kelly was one of the first people to step in and show up. She understood the landscape in a way few people could. She didn't offer platitudes—she offered truth. For privacy reasons, I won't get into details, but Kelly is also a cancer survivor, fighting that battle a few years before I started, so she gets it—she knows exactly what I'm going through. And the thing about Kelly is, she doesn't need credit. She doesn't need fanfare. She just loves you, and if you're lucky enough to be one of the people in her circle, you know that love comes without conditions or expiration dates.

I've said before that I don't know how I'd have made it through parts of my life without Christina, but Kelly is on that same list. She has carried parts of our family that would have otherwise fallen apart. And if there's anything *normal* about my life, it's the extraordinary presence of a sister like her.

Of course, as we all got older, life became more complicated. The easy closeness of childhood began to shift into something less constant but, in some ways, more meaningful. We weren't sharing bedrooms or backyard adventures anymore—we were managing jobs, families, responsibilities, and in my case, a growing list of diagnoses that forced me to see the world, and myself, through a very different lens.

Adam, Kelly, and I all took different paths—emotionally, professionally, geographically—but the roots remained. Kelly and I, especially, found ways to stay connected through it all. As my life took more unexpected turns—through illness, recovery, and reinvention—she never drifted. Our conversations evolved from shared jokes and music into deep talks about survival, identity, and perspective. She became one of the few people I could confide in without explanation or filter.

Adam and I, on the other hand, had a rockier path. The moments that once brought us together started to feel like exceptions instead of habits. What had been automatic became occasional. Maybe it was our differences, or maybe it was how similar we really were that made things hard. We loved each other, but when things went sideways, that love hid itself quickly. His demons looked different than mine, but they came from some of the same places. We both learned how to mask pain in ways that worked—until they didn't. Our relationship has been tested time and again, and while it's never been easy, there's always been love at the core. I'll talk more about that soon.

Andrew, too, became more distant over time, not by choice or desire, but by circumstance. The closeness we had in childhood gave way to adult lives managed by different hands. That loss, to this day, is one of the hardest for me to carry— not because he did anything wrong, but because others in our family did.

That's the thing about growing up—especially in a family like ours. You start to realize that love doesn't always look like greeting cards or group hugs. Sometimes it's showing up in a hospital room. Sometimes it's wiring money when someone's too proud to ask. And sometimes, love looks like a Pearl Jam concert in a smoky Madison bar, when someone lets you feel like you belong, just as you are.

Adulthood has a way of testing even the strongest bonds. But if those bonds were built with love and sacrifice—and in my case, a hell of a lot of forgiveness—they don't break. They stretch. They get quieter. But they're still there, humming beneath the noise of everything else.

And in the chapters ahead, you'll see just how much I've relied on those bonds to get through the darkest moments of my life—and how, sometimes, even the strongest threads can unravel when the weight becomes too much.

INTERLUDE: BMX Bravado

Back in the day, bikes were more than just a way to get around—they were your status symbol. If you had a cool bike, you were cool. And if you were lucky enough to ride something like a Diamondback or a Mongoose, you basically felt like a legend.

I saved and saved, stashing away every dollar I could to buy that street cred. Eventually, I did it—I bought a Diamondback (with some help from my parents). Chrome, slick tires, padded handlebars. It was everything.

With coolness came confidence. And with confidence came a wildly inflated sense of bravery. One day, riding high on my new wheels, I offered to give my buddy Scott a lift home. We called it "doubling"—he'd sit on the handlebars while I pedaled. Not the safest idea, but hey, we were 12. Safety wasn't cool.

Scott hopped up front on the handlebars, facing away from me with his head turned over his shoulder as we rode, chatting the whole way like it was any other afternoon. And then, right in the middle of a sentence, he suddenly turned his head forward, eyes wide.

"Dude... seriously. It's not funny," he said, totally deadpan.

I had no idea what he was talking about.

Until we slammed into the back of a parked car.

I didn't even have time to react. One second, I was pedaling, the next I was airborne—launched over Scott in what felt like slow motion. We both hit the pavement, scraping every inch of exposed skin.

We laid there for a moment, stunned and trying not to cry—because crying wasn't cool either. Then we got up, checked for broken bones, and walked the rest of the way to Scott's house, hoping they owned an industrial-sized box of Band-Aids.

I never doubled anyone again.

At least not until I got those super cool rear pegs installed on the back tire—the ultimate upgrade that let your friends ride in style, without risking facial reconstruction.

CHAPTER 6: Best Friend Lost

I don't remember the exact moment things crossed the line, only the feeling that settled in once they had. Conversations started to trail off instead of ending, phone calls went unanswered, and excuses arrived before questions were asked. Nothing dramatic happened all at once—no explosion, no confrontation—but the air changed. And once it did, it became impossible to pretend that everything was still *normal*.

Adam and I were always close. Closer than most brothers with a four-year age gap probably should've been. Maybe it was the chaos of our house, or the bond that forms when you're both navigating the outside struggles that were a part of our upbringing, but from a young age, we just clicked. He was the older brother I idolized, and for most of our lives, he made me feel like more than just the kid tagging along. He made me feel like I belonged.

We shared a love of music, sports, and sarcastic humor. We made each other laugh when everything else in life felt heavy. Whether it was long drives blasting the Beastie Boys on a cassette radio or hours spent on the basketball court, Adam was always right there—part big brother, part best friend, part co-conspirator. We got each other in a way that only siblings who've grown up under the same roof, with the same dysfunctions, possibly can.

Even as adults, we stayed close. Some of my best memories are from all his visits to Madison when I became a student at the University of Wisconsin. He always joked that he "went to Wisconsin…on the weekends." The post-college years, when we had houses just a few blocks from each other, we'd grab beers, grill out, vent about life, and laugh until our stomachs hurt. And then there was softball—our sacred tradition. We played in an old man recreational league, against an aging group of guys that were deceptively good at this slow-paced sport. It was more than a game—it was a ritual, a time where he and I, along with a big group of our mutual friends, would gather to have a good time and enjoy life.

There never was any doubt that, when the time came, Adam and I would serve as each other's Best Man at our weddings. Our bond was so tight that I don't think either of us actually asked the other—it was correctly assumed. I found my way to the alter a few years before Adam did, so he was the first to turn that life event into an open mic at a comedy club.

As you'll learn later in this memoir, Christina and I met at a young age. I was 17 years old, and she was 16. Adam first met Christina at his college apartment when I brought her with me to a party he was hosting. Traditionally, guests that young would have been turned away, but it was me, so we were welcomed with open arms. Fast-forward to my wedding and of course Adam wasn't going to miss the opportunity to make he and I both sound like creeps. He detailed the evening when he was first introduced to my future bride…

"So, there I am, having a party at my apartment, and Matt brings this 16-year-old girl with him." The reception crowd groaned and I'm certain they missed my rebuttal that I was only

17. The story continued, *"I was like 'Dude, what the hell—she's 16?!?'"* his tone clearly implying that I had done something wrong, before quickly flipping the script. *"Doesn't she have any friends she could have brought with?'"* The roar of laughter was deafening. Adam's personality was on full display. His timing and uncanny knack for dishing it out, while also being willing to take it, was admirable. He never took anything too seriously and enjoyed life to the fullest. It's just who he was.

Then, in his mid-30's, everything changed.

Adam blew out his knee at a softball game, chasing a fly ball in the outfield. For some reason, there was sewer grate hidden in the outfield grass and his cleat got caught as he ran. The leg stopped abruptly, as the rest of his body continued on—that was the moment everything started to unravel. The injury was bad. Surgery followed and then came the painkillers— just a short-term prescription, or so we thought. But those pills—they had claws.

Around the same time, I went under the knife to correct some severe neck pain I was enduring. Doctors discovered a herniated disc in my neck (C5/C6 for those that understand) and determined surgery to be the best course of remediation. Following that procedure, I too was prescribed painkillers to aide in my recovery. I mention this for perspective. Having been handed a bottle of opioids myself, I can fully understand the allure and the grip these drugs can have on an individual, especially someone with an addictive personality. I'd be lying if I said there weren't times where I sought a couple of extra pills from Adam's stash, and he was always willing to share. I look back now and feel grateful that the stranglehold of opioids never fully overwhelmed me. I "had my fun" and then stopped. I wish Adam had done the same.

At first, it didn't seem like a big deal. He was recovering, sore, tired—nothing out of the ordinary. Nothing seemed urgent enough to stop the day from moving forward. That was part of the problem. As the months passed, I noticed the change. He was less present. Flaky. Short-tempered. Our conversations got thinner, our laughs less frequent. He'd cancel plans, disappear for stretches, then reappear like nothing happened. I didn't want to believe it. I couldn't. We were too close. This couldn't be happening to us.

But it was.

Adam had fallen into something dark and relentless, and no matter how much I wanted to pull him out, I couldn't reach him. Opioid addiction doesn't make announcements. It doesn't knock on the door and wait for permission. It creeps in, takes root, and reshapes the person you love into someone you barely recognize.

For years, I had leaned on Adam. In so many ways, he had been one of my safety nets—someone who always knew what to say, who always showed up. But now, he was the one slipping, and I was powerless to catch him. I tried everything I could think of—talking, reasoning, tough love, soft love. Nothing stuck.

The hardest part was watching the distance grow between us. It wasn't sudden—it was slow, like fog creeping in. There were still flashes of the old Adam—the jokes, the random texts about a backyard fire, the moments where it felt like we were back on the softball field again. But they were fewer and farther between. And eventually, they stopped coming at all.

Addiction doesn't just steal a person—it steals your history with them. It takes the trust, the laughter, the shorthand, and replaces it with uncertainty and silence. I missed my brother long before he was gone. I mourned him in real-time, while he was still there.

And yet, I still love him fiercely. Always have. Always will. The bond we had—have—is real. And I still carry hope. Hope that the real Adam is still in there, buried but not broken. Hope that, one day, we'll lace up our cleats again, even if it's just for a game of catch in the backyard. Hope that he knows, even now, that I never gave up on him. Not once.

Because that's what brothers do.

Addiction doesn't happen in a vacuum. When one person falls, the shockwave doesn't stop at their feet—it moves outward, fast and unforgiving, touching everyone who loves them, everyone who remembers who they were before. When Adam fell into addiction, it didn't just take him. It took something from all of us.

At first, we didn't have a name for it. We just knew something felt—off. The late responses. The get-togethers where Adam seemed like he was in another world. The sudden anger that flared up over nothing, followed by days of silence. It was easy to excuse at first—he's tired, he's stressed, work is a lot, the knee surgery took more out of him than expected. But deep down, we knew. Even if we didn't want to say it out loud.

In those moments, my parents never really acknowledged it or talked about it. They had to have known, but they didn't let on. My dad was so busy with work and the pressures of making his business thrive that he may have just missed it all together, but there likely was a hint of denial in there. How could this be? He raised his son better than this. As the years went on, he tried, in his own way, to help the situation, but by that time, Adam was too far gone.

My mom, on the other hand, responded the way she always

had—by trying to fix it. That said, there were multiple sides to her motivation. On one hand, she wanted to help her first-born son, the child she once rocked to sleep, but on the other hand, she wanted to mask what was really going on from the outside world. I think her Catholic guilt fused with a kind of emotional self-preservation. If she admitted how bad things really were, she'd have to face the truth: that Adam was in a freefall. And there was no cushion soft enough to catch him. What would that look like to the family and friends around us? She liked to believe that everyone saw the Saunders' as this picture-perfect family, rooted in religion and faith. Anything outside of that was an embarrassment. Part of me can understand, as my parents suffered for many years, dealing with the stares and judgement of Andrew by uneducated bystanders, but at some point, she needed to realize that every family has their Adam. Maybe it's not addiction, but there are skeletons in every closet. This need to portray the perfect family is why she forced my half-siblings out of our lives years earlier (how could this perfect Catholic family have a divorce and two other children around and still be considered pious?) —it's a pattern that is easy to see now but was difficult to decipher back then.

Kelly and I talked about it often—sometimes too often. We'd rehash conversations, piece together vague texts, try to make sense of the silence. She hated feeling powerless. We both did. Kelly, being who she is, kept trying to include Adam in the world, kept offering invitations, lifelines, moments of connection. But even when he accepted, he just wasn't the same person. Every time, it was another little tear in the fabric of our family.

Holidays became a source of anxiety. Would Adam show up?

Would he be sober if he did? Would someone say the wrong thing? Should we just pretend everything was fine for the sake of keeping the peace? Those unspoken questions hovered over every gathering, thick in the air like humidity before a storm.

Andrew, sweet Andrew, never really understood what was going on—but he felt it. He felt the tension, the missing pieces, the way the room changed when someone brought up Adam's name. He'd ask simple questions that carried impossible weight. *"Why isn't Adam coming?"* and *"Is he mad at us?"* I didn't know how to answer without breaking his heart.

But the hardest part of all was realizing this thing—this addiction—was bigger than any of us. It wasn't a phase or a string of bad decisions. It was a disease. And it had infected not just Adam's body and mind, but our family's dynamic. It turned trust into suspicion. Turned conversations into attempted interventions. Turned love into labor.

We still loved Adam. That never changed. But some of us were tired. Tired of wondering. Tired of waiting. Tired of holding our breath every time the phone rang.

And yet, we kept showing up. Because that's what you do when someone you love disappears into something bigger than either of you. You keep setting a place at the table. You keep hoping they'll walk through the door. You keep loving them—not in the easy way, but in the real way. The hard way.

Deep down, it's the part that haunts me the most. Sharing in those early stages of discovery, when opioids were first introduced to us, I was not the right person to be riding shotgun in that out-of-control vehicle. I could have done more. I should have. I wish I had cut both of us off much sooner. It's not an excuse, but rather an explanation, that when the drugs didn't fully control me and I was able to put them away for good, I assumed Adam would do the same.

During the worst of Adam's addiction, when it felt like everything was coming apart at the seams, I had to make the hardest decision of my life: keep pouring myself into trying to save my brother or step away entirely so I could save myself—and protect my own family.

It was a decision that came slowly, painfully. At first, I tried to do it all. Be the brother who showed up. Be the one making the calls, pushing for treatment, holding family meetings, convincing myself that this time it might stick. But I was also a husband, and a father of three young children who needed me just as much. They were aware of what was going on, Christina at least, and it was taking its toll. Something had to give.

Meanwhile, the addiction was escalating. When Adam was arrested for stealing a prescription pad from his doctor and forging opioid prescriptions, we all believed it might finally be the turning point. Jail time felt like the rock bottom we'd been waiting for—a forced detox, a moment of reckoning, a reset. In this moment, the four of us—my parents, Kelly, and me—met with a therapist to talk through what came next. For the first time, we were aligned. We agreed this was our chance to get Adam real help, and we left that session believing the path forward was finally clear.

That sense of clarity didn't last. Almost as quickly as we found alignment, my mom changed course, convinced she could handle it herself. The plan we had agreed on quietly disappeared, replaced by the familiar instinct to protect, explain, and intervene behind the scenes—this time through a letter she wrote to the judge—filled with emotion and omissions—claiming that Adam was Andrew's full-time caretaker. That if he went to jail, our brother with Down syndrome would suffer. It wasn't true. Adam hadn't been caring for Andrew in any meaningful way for some time. But that letter worked. The court granted Adam a Huber sentence—report to jail at night, but free to come and go during the day. The one real chance we had to get him real help evaporated in the name of keeping him comfortable.

I was crushed. Not just by the lie—but by what it meant.

The letter changed everything. What could have been leverage became leniency, and what felt like a moment for accountability slipped away. Whatever chance we thought we had to force real help dissolved, leaving us back where we started—only now with the added weight of knowing we had been close, and that it was gone. That moment changed so much for me. My mother's denial, her need to protect Adam's image over his actual well-being, was the final barrier. I realized that as long as she protected the fiction, no real change could happen. We weren't helping him—we were helping him hide. And in doing so, we were slowly losing each other.

It was then that I had to face the impossible truth: I couldn't save Adam. No matter how hard I tried, no matter how much I loved him. I had done everything I could think to do, and it still wasn't enough. And the more I tried, the more I was disappearing from the life I had built with Christina, with Alex, Olivia, and Jacob. My kids were still so young. They needed my presence. They needed my strength. They needed all of me—and the only way to give that was to stop giving pieces of myself to a battle I could no longer fight.

So, I chose my family.

Not because I stopped loving Adam. Not because I stopped hoping he'd get better. But because the collateral damage was starting to reach my wife and children, and I couldn't let that happen. I had already spent years sacrificing, trying to save my best friend, but I couldn't willingly sacrifice the people I loved most to the wreckage Adam was creating.

Walking away didn't feel like relief. It felt like grief. I mourned that version of Adam every day. I mourned the brother who used to laugh with me until our ribs hurt, the one who played softball by my side, who knew me better than almost anyone. But that Adam was gone—and the one left behind couldn't see past his pain long enough to let anyone in.

I set boundaries. I stopped taking calls that ended in manipulation or half-truths. I stopped holding out my hand only to watch it get slapped away. I stopped asking how he was doing when I knew I wouldn't get an honest answer.

It was the right choice. But it was also the most heartbreaking.

Christina never judged me for it. She held me through it. And I looked at my kids—at their innocence, their joy, their need for their father—and I knew I had made the only choice I could live with. I would always be Adam's brother. But I had to stop trying to be his savior.

Because I had my own life to live. And more than anything, I owed it to my wife and children not to be pulled under by someone who wasn't ready to be pulled up.

Addiction is a disease. It's easy to get angry at those who are gripped by this affliction, especially when their actions hurt the people around them. You want to believe they can just stop—that if they loved you enough, they would. But it doesn't work that way. Addiction rewires the brain. It buries the person you knew under layers of desperation, denial, and dependence.

I spent years trying to separate my brother from his addiction, clinging to the hope that the man I grew up with was still in there. And maybe he was. But the reality is, until someone chooses recovery—and is truly ready for it—there's only so much anyone on the outside can do. That helplessness is one of the hardest things I've ever faced.

I will always love my brother. But loving someone with addiction means walking a painful line between hope and heartbreak. And sometimes, choosing to protect yourself and your own family doesn't mean you've given up on them. It just means you're trying to survive, too.

If there's a silver lining, it would be this: Adam's addiction has opened my eyes to the dangers and horrors of this disease. I've used this real-world knowledge to inform how I've navigated the past ten years of cancer procedures, specifically limiting, and in some cases declining, pain medications. If truly necessary, I limit them to when I am in-patient and under the care of medical professionals. I don't mention that to make myself sound better, I'm just trying to carve something useful out of the wreckage.

CHAPTER 7: The Intervention That Wasn't

Eventually, the urgency faded. What had felt like a turning point dissolved into long stretches of quiet, and the absence of news became its own answer. That's when it sank in that we were no longer moving toward anything—just forward.

Ultimately, we had failed.

We never pulled it off. Not in the way you see on TV or read about in recovery memoirs—no circle of chairs, no scripted letters, no moment of impact where the addict breaks down in tears and agrees to get help. What we had was more fractured. Less structured. A series of one-off attempts, good intentions, missed signals, and one major opportunity that quietly slipped through our fingers.

But each of us tried. In our own way.

Kelly was in it from the beginning. She was loud when she needed to be, unwavering when others grew tired. She didn't sugarcoat the situation, didn't pretend not to see what was happening. She confronted Adam head-on, called out the behavior, offered support—but only if he was willing to be honest. I admired that in her. I still do. She was fierce in her love, but also willing to hold boundaries. She carried hope and frustration side by side and never gave up, even when her efforts were ignored, twisted, or flat-out rejected.

I wish I could say the same about myself.

I was the quieter one. The observer. Over time, I stayed at a distance, offering passive support—never really pushing hard, never really backing off either. I convinced myself that being the steady, calm presence was enough. I thought: if he wants help, he'll ask for it. I rationalized my inaction, thinking maybe I didn't want to drive him further away. But looking back, I often wonder if what I saw as "support" just looked like avoidance. If my reluctance to get involved was interpreted as indifference. I never stopped caring—but maybe I never made that clear enough.

And then there was my mom.

She was—complicated. She loved Adam more than anyone. Fiercely. Unconditionally. And perhaps, dangerously. She wanted him to be better, but not in a way that exposed the truth. Not in a way that made it real. She wanted to keep the image of her son clean—for herself, for others, maybe even for him. She denied the depth of his addiction, buried the evidence, made excuses, and painted over the truth with layers of hope and delusion. She believed she was protecting him. Maybe she was also protecting herself from the unbearable weight of guilt and helplessness that comes when a mother watches her child slowly disappear.

The closest we came to organizing something formal was when Adam went to jail. That moment was a window—a sliver of time when we could've pulled something together, rallied the people who cared about him, brought in professional help, and tried to reset the course of his life. We thought, for once, the universe had given us a pause button. We began planning. We talked logistics. We wrote things down. For a brief moment, we all aligned.

But then, my mom backed out.

Despite initially agreeing, she unraveled it from the inside. She lied to family members about why Adam had been arrested. She downplayed the severity. She refused to let anyone refer to it as "an addiction." She said he just needed rest, a break, a fresh start. I think, deep down, she couldn't bear to have the image of her son shattered in front of everyone. So, she protected that illusion at all costs—even if it meant throwing away our best and only real shot.

And just like that, it was gone.

No chairs. No confrontation. No reckoning.

The intervention never happened.

And I've thought about it every day since.

Interventions, when done right, aren't just confrontations— they're lifelines. They're expressions of collective love, clarity, and consequence. They say, *"We see you drowning. We're throwing you this rope. Grab it, and we'll pull together."* They don't always work. But sometimes—sometimes they do. Sometimes that's all it takes to shift the story from tragic to redemptive.

Not long after the arrest faded into the background, the calls started sounding the same again. Different circumstances, same concern. That's when it became clear the moment we thought might change everything hadn't. I still believe, with everything in me, that if we had gotten to him at the right time, in the right way, with the right people and the truth fully on the table—it could have changed everything. Maybe not forever. Maybe not completely. But maybe enough. Maybe just enough to interrupt the spiral, to buy some time, to get him through the storm and show him a way out. Maybe enough to save him.

I don't blame any one of us. We all acted out of love. Kelly's version of love was real and raw. Mine was quieter, more restrained. My mom was desperate, tangled in fear and denial. And Adam—Adam was just sick. He needed help. But we never quite got on the same page long enough to give him the chance to take it.

We lost something when that intervention fell apart—not just the opportunity to change Adam's life, but the opportunity to come together, as a family, in truth and action. We let silence win. We let fear win. After that, things between my mom and me were never openly tense—but they weren't the same either. Conversations stayed polite, familiar, and carefully contained, as if we were both avoiding a subject we didn't know how to hold together. Nothing was said, but plenty was understood.

Sometimes I replay it all in my head. I wonder what that moment could have looked like. I picture us gathered— nervous, trembling, tearful. I imagine someone reading a letter, telling Adam how much we love him, how scared we are, how we're not going to let him slip away without a fight. I imagine him sitting quietly, staring at the floor. I imagine that pause, that long, tense moment where he could go either way.

And I let myself imagine him saying yes.

I'll never know how that would have played out.

But I do know this: we were close. Close enough that I will carry the ache of that almost-intervention for the rest of my life.

We wanted to save him. We tried in the only ways we knew how.

But love without action can't always win. And silence doesn't heal sickness.

If we had done it—just once, with unity and honesty and no

more hiding—I truly believe this chapter might have ended very differently.

What I've come to understand is that loving someone doesn't mean you can save them, no matter how clear the path seems or how badly you want it to work. Sometimes all you can do is show up, speak when it matters, and live with what follows when the outcome isn't what you hoped for. That kind of acceptance doesn't bring closure—but it does bring clarity, and for a long time, that has had to be enough.

CHAPTER 8: The Space Between

Life didn't reset after everything that happened, but it did keep moving. I grew older, more independent, and more focused on what came next, even as my relationship with my mom settled into something quieter and more complicated. The urgency was gone, but the weight of what we'd been through together hadn't disappeared—it had just changed shape.

Our relationship had grown complex—close, yes, but layered with expectations, unspoken tensions, and, later in life, some irreconcilable truths. And nothing tested that relationship more than Adam's addiction.

It had been simmering for years—her denial, my frustration, the quiet pain we both carried for very different reasons. But the breaking point came the day she accused me of intentionally excluding Adam from my youngest child's birthday party.

Jake was turning two. Christina and I had planned a small, simple backyard celebration—cake, games, close friends and family. It wasn't meant to be dramatic, just a sweet day for a little boy surrounded by people who loved him. We hadn't sent a formal invite—none were sent, it was that kind of casual gathering—but we assumed, as always, that my mom would pass along the details to Adam, as we had all done for each other a thousand times before. For whatever reason, she decided it *"wasn't her place to invite Adam on my behalf"* and didn't let him know. When I asked if Adam was coming, she said, *"I don't think so. You never invited him."* I was furious, but I bit my tongue and immediately called Adam to let him know. He said he could no longer make it, as he had other plans, but he'd be sure to stop by and drop off Jake's present, since he assumes that's the only reason I was extending the invitation. In that moment, my anger turned to defeat, and I knew this was the beginning of the end.

The next morning, wearing my heart on my sleeve, I stopped by my parents' house to tell them how I was truly feeling. I didn't plan to explode—but I was already holding onto too much for too long. And when my mom met me at the door, shaking her head in disappointment, saying how cruel it was to *"leave Adam out,"* something in me snapped.

The words came hard and fast, sharper than I intended, laced with anger and years of pent-up grief. I said things I wish I hadn't—the kind of words you don't forget, even after apologies. But I also said the truth.

I told her I couldn't keep doing this—pretending everything was okay when it wasn't. I couldn't keep pretending Adam was just a misunderstood guy who'd fallen on hard times. He was an addict. And until she acknowledged that, I couldn't be part of this anymore. I couldn't keep walking into a house where reality was bent to protect one person, while the rest of us were silently unraveling.

I said I was done. That until she stopped choosing denial over her own family's safety, I was stepping away.

I remember her face—shocked, trembling, defensive. I had never spoken to her like that before. My dad stood in the hallway, silent. He didn't interrupt. He didn't correct me. He just looked exhausted. Because he knew I was right. He always did. But he was also her husband, and that put him in a place where truth was a quiet thing—something to acknowledge privately but never act on.

That confrontation wasn't the first time I had tried to get through to her. There had been many. One of the hardest was when I confronted her about Adam spending time alone with my kids—Alex and Olivia—while Christina and I worked. My mom was our childcare lifeline. She helped watch the kids during the week, something we were deeply grateful for. But more than once, I'd show up after work to pick them up, only to find they weren't there. *"They're out with Adam,"* she'd say, as if it were a sweet surprise.

He'd take them out for ice cream or to the park—doing what she saw as fun, uncle things. But when he returned, I could see it in his eyes. He was high. I knew it. The slight slur in his speech, the way his pupils darted around, the way he smiled too much and said too little. It was obvious.

I pulled my mom aside and asked her directly: *"Do you really believe he's sober?"*

"Yes," she said without hesitation. *"He's doing better. He just wants to spend time with his niece and nephew."*

"Would you still say that," I asked, *"if something horrible happened to the kids while he was high?"*

She didn't answer. Not really. She just looked at me with that same tight smile, the one that said, *"let's not go there."* The one that said, *"if I don't admit it, it isn't real."*

But it was real. And it was dangerous.

That was when I started pulling back—mentally, emotionally, physically. I began limiting visits. When Jacob was born, Christina transitioned to a stay-at-home-mom. I stopped sharing updates about Adam's behavior or my concerns because I knew the conversation would go nowhere.

I had made peace with my decision. I wasn't being cold. I was being a father. My children's safety came first. Their peace came first. Christina came first. And I refused to let guilt, tradition, or family pressure cloud that anymore.

Walking away from your family doesn't always look like slamming a door. Sometimes it's a slow fade, a protective retreat. But that fateful day at my parents' house, it was clear, definitive, and painful. I set a boundary. And while I hated how it all came out, I don't regret the substance of what I said.

Because if I didn't say it then, I don't know who I would've become.

My dad later pulled me aside and said, *"You're not wrong."* It was quiet, almost whispered. But it meant the world to me. He knew. He had always known. He just didn't know how to act on it from where he stood. Stuck between a son who was right and a wife who wouldn't bend.

Sometimes the space between love and truth is too wide to bridge. And sometimes, you love people best by stepping away—by no longer playing a part in the lie they've built to survive.

What I didn't know—couldn't have known that day I stood in my parents' doorway unloading years of pain and truth— was that it would be the last real conversation my mother and I would have until many years later.

My decision to walk away wasn't temporary. I had hoped, maybe naively, that things might shift with time. That with distance, perspective would find its way in. That my mom might eventually say, *"I understand now. I know you did what you had to do."* But that day at the door, I didn't just draw a line—I carved a trench.

And she, in turn, pulled away from me too.

Other than two or three brief and emotionally distant encounters over the next sixteen years, we lived separate lives. She was still my mother, but not in the way that counted. Not in the way that comforted. Holidays came and went. Birthdays. Anniversaries. Major surgeries and diagnoses. Milestones for my kids. She wasn't there. Not really. And in her absence, I grieved—not just the relationship we lost, but the one I had once believed we could still have.

My father tried to stay tethered to both sides, but he was caught in an impossible position. He loved us—me, Christina, the grandkids, Kelly and her family—but he also loved his wife. And being her husband often meant staying quiet to keep the peace. It wore on him. I saw it. In his eyes. In his posture. He became a man divided, doing his best to keep his love from fracturing into guilt. I never blamed him for that. I just hated the situation that forced him to choose silence as a coping mechanism.

And then, out of nowhere, life forced my mother and I back into the same room.

Christina and I were at my sister-in-law's cabin, a couple hours north of Milwaukee, when the news came in: my father was in the hospital. It wasn't good. His dementia had wasted his body away to nothing and the end was near. I raced home, adrenaline pushing me faster than I should've been driving. All I wanted was one more moment. One more look. One more I love you.

I was too late.

He was gone.

I walked into that hospital carrying sixteen years of silence and regret. And yet, in that moment, nothing else mattered. Not the arguments. Not the wedge between my mother and me. Not the time lost. All I could feel was grief—and a desperate need to connect with the one person who, no matter what had happened between us, had once held me in her arms and called me son.

So, I walked over to her.

I put everything else aside—every ounce of anger, pain, disappointment. I told her I was sorry for the loss of her husband—my father. I tried, in that moment, to let the past be a conversation for another day and just express my sincere condolences for her loss—our loss. I reached out to hug her, hoping for some kind of reciprocation.

She said nothing.

She turned her back on me.

I stood there, stunned. Still reaching. Still hoping. But she had made her choice.

And in that moment, the space between us became permanent—or so I thought.

CHAPTER 9: Echoes From a Closed Door

There wasn't a final phone call or a definitive fight—other than the profanity-laced "conversation" my mother and I had the day after Jake's 2nd birthday. Just a stretch of time where holidays passed, birthdays went unacknowledged, and conversations that once felt automatic simply stopped happening. At some point, I realized the distance had become the default—and that realization carried more weight than any argument ever could have.

Estrangement is a word we don't say out loud much. It carries too much weight—too much implication. It doesn't sound like a moment or a mistake; it sounds like a condition, a diagnosis, maybe even a failure. But for many families, it's not an anomaly—it's part of the story. And for mine, it has become one of the quieter, more painful truths I've had to learn to live with.

The strange part is, I didn't see it coming. At least not this way.

I've spent a lot of time thinking about estrangement as something that happens *to* you. Someone pulls away, stops calling, builds walls. But in my case, I was the one who faded. The one who became the distant one. Not out of anger or pride, but out of exhaustion. Out of pain. Out of a deep need to protect whatever small pieces of *normal* I had left.

Somewhere along the line, I stopped trying. Not with everyone, but with enough people that it shows. With everyone *but* Kelly, really. She's the one person who's been constant—the one thread of connection I've managed to hold on to while the rest of the fabric has frayed.

And that fraying has taken a toll in ways I didn't anticipate. One of the most heartbreaking outcomes of this widening divide is the distance it's created between me and my brother Andrew. We were never at odds. But sometimes, a divide with one person means you're inevitably pulled away from another. The rift between my mother and me—complex, unresolved, and full of years of silence and sidestepping—has acted like a fault line. And Andrew, through no real fault of his own, stands on the other side.

Andrew didn't do anything wrong. He didn't contribute to the tension or the history or the heartbreak. But because he has Down syndrome and lives with my mom full-time, he became part of what I had to leave behind. And that—out of everything—has been the most devastating part of this estrangement.

There's an innocence to Andrew—a light. His love is pure and uncomplicated. He doesn't play games or hold grudges. He doesn't calculate or judge. He just *is*. And the bond we've shared over the years has always been one of the purest, most joyful parts of my life.

But the rift between me and my mother created an unavoidable wall. There was no path to see him that didn't lead through her. And over time, it became too hard. Too messy. Too painful.

Andrew—sweet Andrew—he just wants to be loved. To laugh. To hug. To be included. The fact that I've missed out on so much of his life—birthdays, celebrations, even just the day-to-day stuff—it breaks me in ways I don't know how to describe.

In a strange and deeply unfair way, my brother has become collateral damage in a war he didn't start. And the guilt of that sits heavy on my chest every single day.

Kelly has remained a constant in all of this—my sister, my sounding board, my lifeline. She understood why I pulled away, maybe because she's seen firsthand how deep some of those wounds go. But even she can't undo the ripple effects. Even she can't bridge the distance I feel from the rest of my family.

What I've come to understand is that even when you're not the underlying cause of the fracture, you can still end up carrying the ache of it. You can still be the one left feeling the weight of everything unsaid, everything unresolved. And for me, that ache is no longer a passing discomfort. It's permanent.

I used to tell myself there was time. That maybe things would come around. That wounds would close and people would soften. But time doesn't feel infinite anymore. I live in Florida now—over 1,000 miles from where those reconnections would even be possible. And beyond that, I'm sick. The kind of sick that makes you calculate your energy, your effort, your emotional bandwidth. The kind of sick that makes you think in terms of "what's left" rather than "what's next."

I no longer believe in the idea that a last-minute reconciliation will appear like a scene from a movie. I don't hold space for a surprise phone call or a tearful reunion. I think, more than anything, I've accepted that whatever healing might have happened, it probably won't. And in that way, this form of estrangement feels more like a death than a falling-out. One I'm grieving, even though almost everyone is still alive.

There's guilt in that. I wonder if I gave up too soon. If I should have fought harder. If the door I quietly closed will stay shut forever. And then there's the other voice—the one that reminds me why I stepped back in the first place. The burnout. The heartache. The toll it was taking on me, at a time when I was already running out of reserves. I was trying to survive. And maybe survival required stepping away.

I don't write this as an excuse. I write it because it's part of the truth. And if this book is anything, it's an attempt to lay all the pieces out there—even the messy ones.

I think about the people I've grown distant from more than they probably realize. I don't wish them ill. In fact, I hope they're doing well. I hope life has brought them peace and joy. But I don't know if they'll ever know that. That's what estrangement does—it replaces knowing with wondering.

And yet, even in that wondering, there's still something else: acceptance. Not the tidy kind, not the kind wrapped in bows. But the kind that settles in after years of hoping something might change. The kind that lets you breathe again, even if it leaves a small hollow in your chest.

I hope anyone reading this who has been on either side of estrangement knows they're not alone. That sometimes, stepping back isn't abandonment—it's self-preservation. That sometimes, love remains even when contact doesn't. And that not every broken thing can be fixed—but that doesn't mean it wasn't once beautiful.

I don't know how much time I have left. I don't say that for sympathy; I say it as a fact. And in this chapter of my life, the one marked by vulnerability and honesty, I feel compelled to say the quiet part out loud: I wish things had turned out differently. I wish the space between us had felt like something temporary, not permanent.

But here I am, with the people who *did* show up. With those who never left. With the small, strong circle that still surrounds me. And for all the people I no longer speak to, I'll just say this—whatever happened, I hope you know I loved you. And maybe that's the truest thing I can leave behind.

INTERLUDE: Two Large Chocolate

After that infamous encounter at the hospital—where my mother turned her back on me just moments after my father passed away—I needed a reset. I decided to get Andrew out of there and take him for lunch. Not surprisingly, his restaurant of choice was Culver's.

Dan, Kelly's amazing husband and Andrew's ride for the day, joined us. The three of us sat at the table, eating our *very* healthy lunches, catching up and trying to bring a little light into an otherwise heavy day.

Once the food was gone, Andrew asked the question I knew was coming.

"Uh, Mattress. You buy me a Concrete Mixer?"

"Of course! What do you want?" I replied.

"Two large chocolate."

Naturally.

I knew full well that if my mom found out Andrew ate two large Concrete Mixers in one sitting, she'd absolutely lose it. And I didn't need to give her another reason to be mad at me. So, I did what any loving brother would do—I tried to bargain.

"How about just one this time?"

"Come on, Mattress. I have two, please?"

I had a plan.

"Okay, two," I said, with a smile.

I walked up to the counter and ordered two *small* chocolate Concrete Mixers—confident I could pull one over on him. They'd still be plenty—just a little less of a sugar bomb. I returned to the table and waited.

A few minutes later, the server appeared, carrying the two mixers on a tray.

The moment Andrew saw them, his face dropped.

He looked at me, shook his head, and said flatly, *"I don't want these. I like large."*

"But there's two," I tried. *"It's the same amount!"*

"Uh, no... I'm okay."

He refused to eat them. Wouldn't even take them home. So, I packed them up, tossed them in my car, and brought them home for my kids. By the time I got there, they were soup.

Andrew lives for routine. He's structured, predictable, and honest to a fault. He'll always appreciate the gesture, but if it's not what he asked for, he's going to let you know.

And honestly? I love that about him.

CHAPTER 10: Saying Goodbye

When I was first diagnosed, my phone didn't stop buzzing. Texts, calls, messages from people checking in, offering help, asking what I needed. I remember sitting there, overwhelmed by the support, grateful for it—and noticing, even then, the one silence that felt louder than all the rest.

Cancer had invaded our lives as early as Christina's scare in 2014 (more on that in a bit), and when I was officially diagnosed in January of 2016, the outpouring of support from family and friends was overwhelming and humbling. I knew I was surrounded by an extraordinary support group, but nothing prepared me for how remarkable my inner circle truly was—and still is.

Curiously absent from that group was the one person you'd assume would never let anything get in the way of reaching out to support someone dealt this awful news. No matter the circumstances of our broken relationship, cancer would certainly eclipse all of that and, in a weird way, become the healing moment that could reunite a mother and son.

In the days that followed, I kept expecting my phone to ring with her name on it. Each time it didn't, I told myself it was still early, that she'd call when she was ready. Days passed, then weeks, and the silence slowly stopped feeling accidental.

Admittedly, I didn't actively reach out to my mom to let her know the news—a decision I quickly saw as selfish and short-sighted on my part. But I wouldn't say it came from spite. The chaos of the situation left me thinking more about next steps than who needed to know. Besides, our community was small and tight knit. Surely the news would filter down to my parents before I could even make that call.

Which is exactly what happened for my father.

Before I had a chance to reach out, he called me to check in, to ask if there was anything I needed or anything he could do. I remember that phone call vividly. The two of us shared a cry, with an overarching plea to stay strong and persevere. My dad asked, knowing the existing rift, whether he could share the news with my mother. Of course, I told him he could.

Months later, I would learn that he had—but not before someone else beat him to it. I didn't hear it from her. I learned later, through someone else, in a way that felt almost incidental—like a detail that slipped out when it wasn't supposed to. I remember sitting with that information, trying to understand how something so significant could reach her without ever making its way back to me.

As I understand it, the news was inadvertently shared by another Special Olympics family, who stopped my mom at an event to express their support. Rather than being shocked or upset about my diagnosis, my mother flipped the switch to anger. Not anger about the devastating news—but because she had been "embarrassed" in front of her friends. She was upset that she "looked stupid" not knowing. Again—patterns.

That said, I take full responsibility for my decision not to call her directly. In hindsight, I should have put all else aside and picked up the phone. But I didn't. I regret that choice, but

I've also come to terms with it—especially knowing how my mother decided to deal with the news once she had it.

No matter how the message got to her, it was her reaction—or better said, her lack of action—that truly revealed her character. Like so many other times in our lives, my mother chose anger and vindictiveness over grace. If I wasn't going to call her directly, then she wasn't going to acknowledge that I was sick.

Years later, I would learn she was aware of both of my diagnoses. And it breaks my heart to know she never once—not a single time—reached out to show even a small amount of love or support. Instead, she fell back into her favorite role: the victim, the martyr. A role she had spent years perfecting.

It wasn't until my father's funeral—and a couple of in-person and phone conversations—that my mom and I had a chance to talk about my health. She asked questions. I filled her in with details. She expressed remorse for what I was going through. And for a moment, it felt good to bring her in, to feel a flicker of the love she used to provide.

But that moment was short-lived.

She once again denied that she had ever known I had cancer. She said it calmly, without hesitation, as if it were simply a fact: that she hadn't known. I remember the pause that followed, the space where I understood there was nothing left to clarify. In that moment, the silence, the denial, and the years of distance all lined up, and I knew this wasn't a misunderstanding—it was the end. She told me, *"I never reached out because I didn't know,"* which I knew was a lie. And in that moment, the weight of it all—the silence, the denial, the rewriting of truth—crashed over me. I realized this truly was the end. Our already fractured relationship was officially broken beyond repair. The door closed harder than it needed to—not a slam, just firm enough that I knew the conversation wasn't going anywhere else.

I told her that Christina, Olivia, Jacob, and I were moving to Florida—news we both knew meant we would likely never see each other again. One of us will see the other for the last time at one of our funerals.

And that's the kind of silence you never quite get used to.

INTERLUDE: Faith, Or Something Like It

I was raised Catholic—which, in my family, didn't just mean going to church on Sundays. It meant showing up. It meant guilt before grace, appearances before honesty, and above all, it meant keeping up the illusion that everything was fine, even when it very much wasn't.

As a kid, faith felt like part of the furniture—always there, always expected, something you dusted off and sat politely with every Sunday. I didn't question it much. I knelt when I was told, recited the prayers, tried not to laugh during the "peace be with you" handshake. It was just what we did.

But somewhere along the way—maybe when I watched my parents lie to protect an image, maybe when Andrew was stared at by so-called "good Catholics," or maybe when I started watching my own body betray me—I began to wonder what faith was really supposed to be.

Is it supposed to hurt like this? Is it supposed to shame you into silence? Should it feel like something you have to fight to belong to?

When I got sick—really sick—I didn't run to church. I didn't light a candle and beg. I didn't even really pray in the traditional sense. But I *did* start noticing the sacred again. In the way Christina held my hand during treatment. In the way my kids looked at me like I was still their superhero, even when I could barely walk. In the laughter that came at the weirdest, darkest times.

Maybe that's faith. Or maybe it's just the quiet kind of hope that refuses to die, even when everything else seems like it might.

But then—something happened.

At my lowest—when I had all but lost faith, when I wasn't sure what I believed anymore—a renewed spirit showed up out of nowhere. A friend called to tell me that the church near our house was hosting an Anointing of the Sick sacrament. No pressure, she said, but she wanted me to know.

I was reluctant. I hadn't been to church in a long time, and it felt almost hypocritical to race back there now, like I was only showing up because things had gotten bad. But something told me to go. So, I did.

I wasn't sure what to expect. I walked in feeling cautious, skeptical even—but what I found was peace.

The room was full—some familiar faces, but mostly strangers. People had brought their loved ones, their ailing parents, their sick spouses. No one spoke much. There was a quiet reverence to the space. When the priest began moving through the rows, performing the rite—placing oil on our foreheads, offering the blessing—I was overcome.

Everyone participated. No hesitation. Just shared presence, shared vulnerability. And when it was my turn, when the priest placed his hand on my head and I felt the warmth of that moment, I broke down. Not because I was suddenly healed or had all the answers. But because for the first time in a long time, I felt the love *flowing through me*.

Not judgment. Not doctrine. Not the weight of guilt or performance.

Just love.

And for a moment, that was enough.

I don't know if I believe in the church the same way I once did. But I believe in what happened that day. I believe in showing up for each other. I believe in quiet rooms filled with strangers and grace.

I believe in my family. I believe in second chances. I believe in people like Christina, who always shows up for the hard parts. And if that's not faith, I don't know what is.

. . .

In My Given Life, I learned that what we call "normal" is often just what we've grown used to — even when it hurts. Sometimes, it's inherited before it's ever chosen.

II

My Chosen Life

CHAPTER 11: We Were Just Kids

Sitting here now, with more years behind me than ahead, I can't help but smile when I think about how it all began.

Chrissie.

For those that know us well, that might sound odd, but that's how I knew her when we first met, so that's how I wanted to begin this journey through the amazing life she has given me.

Given where we are in life now, I find myself thinking back fondly to how it all began. The twists and turns have been nothing short of eventful, and honestly, if I had the chance to do it all over again, I wouldn't want anything to change. Chrissie has been one of the few constants in my 51-year existence that I've always been so grateful for, and I thank God that He brought her into my world. Of course, our three beautiful children have added to this remarkable life we've built—but it all started with that adorable, blonde-haired cutie I fell head-over-heels for more than 30 years ago.

It's funny to think back on our days at St. Margaret Mary. There we were, literally one room apart for eight years. Her cousin Johnny and I were close friends, but even with all those connections, we somehow never "officially" met. We likely passed each other in the halls, saw each other on the playground, lined up near each other for Christmas chorus concerts. We even spent a whole school year rehearsing for *The Wizard of Oz*—same production, same school—but the stars never aligned.

Then I left, heading downtown to a parochial high school, while she stayed close to home. The distance between us grew even more. I know now I was at her house a few times to swim with Johnny, or to drop Andrew off at Boy Scout meetings— never realizing that his scout leader was my future father-in-law. So close, yet still not quite there.

Thankfully, Milwaukee is a small town in all the best ways. Eventually, the stars did align.

Although I can't remember the first time I saw her at my dad's Mobil station—probably gassing up on her way to a waitressing shift at the Ground Round—I do remember being struck by how beautiful she was. I hoped I'd get the chance to talk to her. As time went on, those short exchanges while she paid for gas turned into brief but meaningful conversations. I'd see her out at the pump and get butterflies, knowing she'd be inside soon. If there was a line of people, I'd silently curse it, because it meant our time would be cut short. I was always embarrassed to be wearing those dorky shop pants and my Mayfair Mobil button-down, but the moments when she was the only customer in the store? I lived for those.

I guess I should be grateful that paying at the pump wasn't a thing yet.

And then it happened—her car overheated. Luckily for both of us, she pulled into the station. I didn't see her drive in, but I'll never forget her walking into the store and asking to use the phone. She needed a ride home. I'll admit I wasn't exactly rooting for her to be stranded, but when it looked like no one was coming to help, I was kind of relieved. I mustered up every ounce of courage I had and offered her a ride after my shift. She said yes. Not only that, but she stuck around while I closed up the shop. It was the longest we'd ever spent together, and I was nervously excited the entire time.

Her house was only a couple miles away, but that ride felt like an eternity—in the best way. I don't remember what we talked about, but I must not have made too big a fool of myself because when I dropped her off, I was already thinking about how to ask her out.

A day or two passed, and I still hadn't worked up the nerve. Finally, my brother mentioned he was throwing a small get-together at his East Side apartment. I decided that was my shot. I dug out an old STMM family directory, found her parents' number, and dialed. I hadn't rehearsed anything. When she picked up, I panicked a little—but I got the words out. And she said yes.

I hung up and smiled like an idiot. The girl I'd been nervously talking to at the gas station for months had agreed to go out with me. It wasn't the fanciest date, but it was a start.

That night finally arrived. I picked her up from the same spot I'd dropped her off just days earlier. I'm sure I was rambling, but the excitement carried me. The party itself was nothing special, but the energy between us was electric. A glance across the room. A hand resting on mine. Sitting on the floor together, fingers slowly intertwining. Then, she stood in front of me, facing away as we talked to someone. She leaned back. I wrapped my arm around her waist. When the room cleared out, I spun her around, we locked eyes—and kissed.

I couldn't believe it.

She might read this and wonder why I was so giddy. But she must understand—I wasn't the guy who had girls chasing after him. I was the funny friend, the guy on the sidelines. The fact that *she* liked *me*? It was the most incredible feeling.

That night was just the beginning. The first summer we spent together was unforgettable. We were inseparable. Every day together felt like something out of a movie. I was excited about college, sure—but nothing compared to how I felt about her. That summer shaped everything.

Before I go further, I have to be honest. I do have one regret.

When we were together that summer, I was on cloud nine. But I had never been in a real relationship before—not like this. And when I moved to Madison that Fall, suddenly we had to be "long-distance." That scared me. I didn't know how to do that. I wasn't mature enough to understand that a relationship doesn't have to end just because it changes. So, I made a stupid, selfish decision: I broke up with her.

It was never about not loving her. I was just too immature to know how to hold on. That's something I've always regretted.

I spent that year in Madison learning how to be on my own. College felt different. My dorm room smelled like instant ramen and stale beer. Bunk beds, a desk cluttered with notes I never read, and a window that looked out over a parking lot. At night, I'd lie there staring at the ceiling tiles, listening to laughter from the hallway and enjoying my independence. I had fun, sure, but not in a way that filled the space she left. I didn't date anyone seriously. I couldn't. I still thought about her all the time. But I also assumed I'd hurt her too much and figured she'd moved on.

Then came the summer. I was back in Milwaukee, working as many shifts at Mayfair Mobil as I could—trying to stay busy. Chicken Fest, the annual neighborhood party filled with locals, rolled around, and although I had to work late, my brother called and begged me to swing by afterward. I was hesitant, but something told me to go.

Thank God I did.

As soon as I walked in and spotted him, there she was—Chrissie. She rushed over and wrapped her arms around me. All the butterflies came back. She was genuinely happy to see me, and I felt the same way. We talked. We reconnected. Just like that, it was as if no time had passed.

From that moment on, we were back together. Every day. Every night. Like we'd never been apart. And we've never been apart since.

Sometimes I wonder—if I hadn't gone to Chicken Fest that night, would we have reconnected? But deep down, I know we would have. It was meant to be.

She could've gone to college somewhere else. She could've left Milwaukee. A thousand different things could've taken her away. But she didn't leave. And I'm forever grateful that we found our way back to each other.

INTERLUDE: Higher Education Begins with a Buzz

The day I was leaving for college, I had all my stuff packed into the truck I borrowed from my cousin, ready to begin what I hoped would be the greatest adventure of my life. One of my first stops was to pick up Dan—my high school buddy and future college roommate. In the excitement of this next chapter, I could feel something wasn't quite right. Dan was quiet. The mood was tense. At first, I figured it was just the emotional weight of him saying goodbye to his parents.

Turns out, it wasn't just that.

A few minutes later, Dan's mom pulled me aside. She looked anxious and deeply distressed. *"We found bottles of liquor in Dan's bag last night,"* she said. *"Apparently someone he worked with at the cemetery—someone of legal age—bought it for him. We talked about it, and I just wanted you to know what's going on. I'll understand if you don't want to live with Dan this year."*

She was completely serious. Her voice full of genuine concern.

And I—well, I had to physically stop myself from laughing out loud.

Because in my head, I wasn't thinking about how this changed anything. I was thinking, *"This is exactly why I want to live with Dan."*

We threw Dan's stuff in the truck and hit the road. The 90-minute drive to Madison was a nonstop string of laughter. Nervous excitement. Stupid jokes. Wild speculation about what our new dorm would look like, how we'd find the best parties, and how we were *definitely* going to be more responsible than people gave us credit for.

Both sets of parents arrived shortly after we did. We made quick work of hauling our boxes and bags into our new digs, all while carefully avoiding the discovery of the *other* bottles—mine—that I had stashed away in my own things. Everyone was in move-in mode: hangers, sheets, awkward parental goodbyes, and well-meaning reminders to study hard and call home occasionally.

We smiled. We nodded. We promised.

And as soon as the door closed behind them, Dan and I made eye contact, grinned like kids on Christmas morning, and immediately mixed up our first dorm room cocktails. They were probably terrible. They were definitely warm. But they were ours—and they marked the beginning of what would become a five-year bender on the campus of the University of Wisconsin.

We didn't know it at the time, but that moment—that combination of freedom, friendship, and just enough rebellion to feel alive—was the start of something unforgettable. College, in all its ridiculous, messy glory, had officially begun.

CHAPTER 12: 2gether 4ever

After high school graduation and the summer we reconnected, Christina enrolled in a travel academy in downtown Milwaukee, where she learned the necessary skills to become a corporate travel agent. School kept her in Milwaukee a little bit longer, but by then I had the maturity to understand that our love was stronger than a 75-mile distance. By Thursday afternoons, I'd stop pretending to pay attention in class, checking the clock every few minutes and replaying the drive from Milwaukee in my head, knowing she was somewhere on the road toward me. All those butterflies I keep talking about were in full flight every time I knew she was coming.

We had so much fun! Parties at my place or at a friend's, somehow sneaking into the bars before we were 21, or just hanging out and being together. We finally had everything we wanted. I'll forever cherish those years. Sure, we did a lot of dumb shit too, but it was all worth it. I can't imagine what my college experience would've been like without her. I appreciated every mile she drove just to spend time with me.

This time around, I wasn't going to mess it up.

I knew in my heart I had found the girl I wanted to spend the rest of my life with. I didn't have much money—whatever I made usually went toward school, partying or food—but I wanted to show her how much I loved her. I made plans to take her out to dinner a few days before Christmas so I could give her a gift early.

Olive Garden was the fanciest place I could afford, but I knew she wouldn't care. I sat there nervously through dinner, with a ring box wrapped in my pocket, trying to work up the courage to ask her the biggest question of my life. When we finished eating, I told her I had two presents. I handed her one small box, which she unwrapped to find a modest piece of jewelry I had picked out. Being the amazing person she is, she smiled and said how much she loved it—even though I could tell she was curious about the second gift.

That's when I looked her in the eyes and nervously asked her to marry me.

Now, I don't know how it usually goes for most guys, but she said *"YES"* so fast and so confidently, I barely had time to finish the sentence. I was ecstatic—and relieved.

Looking back, I realize I didn't exactly follow the "traditional" proposal script. I hadn't saved for an extravagant ring (and to be honest, I'm still a little embarrassed by how little it cost). I didn't ask her father for permission. I didn't plan some big, elaborate moment. But this was all new to me, and I simply followed what felt right. And asking Christina to spend her life with me felt exactly right.

She finished travel school and began her career, knowing exactly what she wanted—and where she wanted to be. I was ecstatic when she joined me in Madison. I finally had what I was missing my freshman year—her. And we got to spend all our time together.

To a certain extent, I miss those days—but everything that followed only got better with each passing year.

INTERLUDE: Rosie Doesn't Even Live Here

Our college crew was close. These weren't just friends—they were family. We did everything together. And when Christina got her own off-campus apartment with a roommate, it became less of a home base and more of a communal living space. For a few of us, it basically felt like we had two places to live.

One frequent fixture was our buddy, Patrick (Rosie to everyone who knows him). After a typical night of college-level "hydration," Rosie often ended up crashing on Christina's couch. It was kind of an unspoken agreement—no questions asked.

One night, well past 2 a.m., Christina and her roommate were startled awake by frantic banging at the front door. Still half-asleep, they shuffled their way to the entry, slippers scraping the wood floor, and called out, *"Who is it?"*

A slurred but confident voice replied, *"Rosie."*

They opened the door to find him standing there, clearly having had more than a few drinks, looking indignant.

"You locked me out!" he announced.

Christina, groggy and confused, blinked a few times and responded, *"You don't even live here!"*

That line became legendary. It was retold for years at weddings, reunions, group texts—it never got old. And no matter how many times we heard it, it only got funnier.

CHAPTER 13: Two Become One

Standing at the back of the church, surrounded by suits, flowers, and nervous energy, I realized this day had finally arrived.

If I thought I was nervous to call Christina (as she's now known) the first time, you can imagine how I felt on September 13, 1997. I mean, I was excited—absolutely—but when the day arrived, I was sweating bullets. Maybe it was the fact that all eyes would be on us for the next 12 hours. Maybe it was the irrational fear that she could change her mind at the last minute. Or maybe—just maybe—it was that illusory ex-boyfriend who'd come bursting through the church doors to object and sweep her away. (Okay, that last one wasn't actually a thought, but you get it.)

Whatever it was, it felt very real. Thankfully, I made it down the aisle without fainting or tripping over my own feet.

I got into position next to my groomsmen and turned to look toward the church entrance. I was holding it together fairly well—until the music changed. That's when the rush hit me. She was about to walk through those doors. The entire crowd shifted slightly, a ripple of energy moving through the pews. And then it happened. There she was—Christina—her arm tucked into her father's, standing in the doorway, radiant and ready to walk toward me.

I was speechless.

Christina looked absolutely stunning. I've always thought she was beautiful, but in that moment, she completely took my breath away. And then it hit me—this was it. I was going to marry her. And I couldn't stop smiling.

Her walk down the aisle felt like it lasted forever, and I loved every single second of it. She looked so happy—so ready. When her dad shook my hand and placed her arm in mine, something clicked. That was the moment. We weren't just "us" anymore—we were one.

The reception that followed was equal parts magical and exhausting. But one thing I never told Christina about that night: every time we were apart—even briefly—I kept looking over at her in disbelief. I couldn't believe she was my wife. And while we laugh about it now, I'm truly glad our wedding song was as long as it was. I could've danced with her forever.

The more I reflect on that day, the more I realize how incredible our journey to that point really was. We were already inseparable before we tied the knot—but now it was official. Some guys joke about marriage like it's a trap, but I loved the idea of being with her all the time. I wouldn't have asked her to be my wife if I didn't plan to enjoy the rest of my life with her by my side.

In some unfiltered (read: alcohol-assisted) conversations with friends over the years, they've admitted their jealousy— not in a mean-spirited way, but in that sincere, confessional way guys sometimes get. Christina was the one they all wanted to hang out with. She was the one they included like she was "one of the guys." She was the one some of them quietly crushed on. And there I was—the guy who got to marry her.

I'm not sure how I got so lucky. But I did.

INTERLUDE: Escape From St. Germain

Before Christina's parents officially became my in-laws, they graciously included me on their annual family trips to northern Wisconsin—usually a blend of camping, swimming, and lazy days in the sun. One summer, I was 18 and Christina was 17. I had spent the week leading up to our trip in nearby Park Falls with my cousins, Dave and Jeff, which almost certainly involved a blur of small-town mischief and late-night shenanigans. At the end of that week, Dave and Jeff agreed to drive me the couple of hours to meet up with Christina and her family in St. Germain.

The plan was simple: they'd drop me off, maybe stay the night at the campground, and head home the next day. But since Jeff and I were 18-year-olds with questionable judgment and some leftover Park Falls energy, we made a pit stop to stock up on a cooler's worth of "adult beverages," figuring we'd wait for the grownups to call it a night before heading to a nearby beach to drink under the stars.

Once we were confident the coast was clear, the four of us—me, Dave, Jeff, and Christina—snuck off to the lake. We were sipping our beers, laughing, and enjoying the stillness of the night when Christina's younger brother and a few of his buddies showed up uninvited, blasting fireworks like they were recreating the Fourth of July. We were less concerned about their antics and more about the attention they might draw. And sure enough, it didn't take long before flashlights appeared on a nearby trail. Park rangers.

Now, if you've never been busted at a Northwoods beach with contraband in your cooler, let me tell you—your instincts kick in fast. Ours told us to run. So, we did. Through thick woods, dodging branches, stumbling down paths in the pitch dark like a scene from *The Blair Witch Project*. When we finally burst through the trees and made it back to the campsite, hearts pounding, we realized one of us was missing.

Jeff.

To be clear, Jeff isn't just any cousin. We're the same age, just a few months apart, and for years we've claimed we're twins who don't look alike—bound by immature humor, poor decision-making, and an uncanny ability to find ourselves in absurd situations. So naturally, panic set in.

After a few minutes of tense whisper-debating, we headed back to look for him. As we crept down the main road, a blinding spotlight hit us square in the face. The ranger. And there, standing sheepishly beside him, was Jeff. The officer explained he had been found alone in the woods. I pulled Jeff aside and whispered, *"What happened?"*

Between embarrassed chuckles, he told me he was sprinting through the dark when he ran full speed into a tree. He was stunned, lying flat on his back, when the ranger's flashlight landed on him. And in true Jeff fashion, when the ranger asked what the hell he was doing, Jeff—dazed and committed to the bit—started gnawing on the tree and muttered, *"What? I'm a beaver."*

The ranger was not amused. It was probably that one-liner that sealed our fate that night. The officers wrote us up for underage drinking, and Dave, who was actually 22, got a citation by association. But we weren't done yet.

What we hadn't considered was that Christina was only 17. Which meant they had to wake up her parents.

I wanted to disappear. I couldn't even begin to imagine what her parents must have been thinking as they were roused from their peaceful sleep to learn their daughter had been drinking beer on a beach and then literally ran into the law—with *me*. Let's just say the rest of the trip was a little tense.

Now, we all laugh about that night. Even Christina's family chuckles when the story comes up. But in that moment, I was absolutely mortified. I wasn't just worried about the ticket—I was genuinely afraid her parents were going to forbid her from seeing me again. In my head, I kept replaying her mom saying, *"You need to find someone more responsible,"* while I stood there covered in pine needles and shame.

It's wild what you survive at 18. And it's even wilder what becomes a cherished—if not slightly cringeworthy—memory.

CHAPTER 14: And Then There Were Three

There we were, starting our lives as Mr. and Mrs., settling into our first official apartment together. It was more than we'd ever had in Madison—two bedrooms and a loft, laundry tucked inside the apartment, and a small balcony that looked out over the Menomonee Falls neighborhood we were starting to call home.

Just like all the milestones in our relationship, I didn't know exactly what I was doing, but I knew I wanted to do it with Christina by my side. I loved our place—even though the furniture was a little sketchy—but early on I think we both felt like something was missing. We knew we wanted to start a family and have kids while we were still young. It was exciting to think about, and surprisingly, it didn't make me nervous at all. I knew she would be an incredible mother, and I would learn how to be a great parent by following her lead.

I never thought I would be as emotional or excited about anything as I was when we got married, but when we found out Christina was pregnant for the first time, my excitement reached a whole new level. She took the test on her own and told me later, and when she did, we were standing in our apartment, just the two of us. I don't remember much of what was said, only the stillness of that moment and the realization that everything we'd been imagining was actually happening. We were going to be parents! And in that moment, it got real—we were bringing a child into the world. Would it be a boy or a girl? Will everything go okay with Christina and the baby? What will we name him or her? So many questions, and seemingly an endless wait until the delivery date. I also remember a conversation we had where we asked the categorically hard-hitting question of, *"What if our baby isn't cute?"* I'm sure it's something that most first-time parents think about at some point, but I felt confident that with Christina as the mother, our child(ren) would be adorable. Spoiler alert: I was right.

The months that followed, and the many doctor appointments that came with them, seemed to take forever. I knew there wasn't anything I could do to speed things up, and it didn't make the wait any easier. I tried to occupy my time with work and getting things ready for our new arrival, but when we purchased the crib, I just couldn't contain myself anymore. I don't remember exactly how early I set it up, but I'm pretty sure the baby room was organized and ready at least three months before we went to the hospital. During those months, I would stop in that room from time to time and just look at everything, imagining what it was going to be like when we had our child in that crib. I think I knew it would be a lot of work, but I didn't care—I was ready.

Then the big day started to draw near. People had told us not to bother packing bags for the hospital in advance, saying it would give us something to do while timing contractions. Ironically, that was the one thing we didn't do early—and, of course, we probably should have. I'm not a deep sleeper, but for some reason, that night I was out cold. I still feel bad that I didn't hear Christina calling for me, but eventually she came just far enough into the bedroom to wake me and let me know her water had broken, leaving a puddle in the bathroom. Honestly, I can't believe I didn't jump out of bed and spring into action. For some reason, I was moving kind of slow. As I sat at the end of the bed putting on my shoes, she called out again to ask what I was doing. *"I'm putting on my shoes, so I don't step in the water."* Again, I'm not sure what I was thinking, but apparently, I didn't want to have wet socks.

We threw together a bag, loaded the car, and slid her carefully into the front seat. I remember how nervous she was about every bump in the road, since the baby was no longer cushioned in amniotic fluid. And the roads between our apartment and the hospital were not exactly smooth. I did my best, but the city of Milwaukee made it tough.

We made it safely and quickly, but as it turned out, there was no real rush. Our impending arrival was not in as much of a hurry as we were. Hours of waiting and labor followed. The baby crowned and went back in. Then crowned again and went back in again. Those minutes felt like hours as we waited to meet our bundle of joy. I can't begin to imagine what it must have been like for Christina. At the time, I really didn't think it was possible to love her more than I already did, but when our son finally made his full entrance into the world, I found myself in complete awe of her. The pain and strength she had to endure for hours, and all I could do was stand there and wait. She proved how strong she was that day, which would be a precursor to the strength she would show throughout our life together.

There he was. Alex Matthew was finally here, and he was the

most beautiful baby I had ever seen. Full disclosure: I never really thought babies were cute before, but that all changed in an instant. He was absolutely perfect. And yes, I know we stressed out about the cone he temporarily formed on his head during his seesaw journey through the birth canal, but none of that mattered. Our family of two was now three, and I was the proudest father in the world. I had two of the most adorable people on this earth in my life, and I felt so lucky to call them my wife and my son. (Side note…the cone went away quickly, and Alex has a perfectly shaped head.)

Our lives had just taken a huge leap—and yet, it was just the beginning. We'd share this same journey two more times, and it never got any less exciting or emotional.

The following months and years were a whirlwind. Alex was the first grandchild on either side, and he received more attention than any child could expect. Visits from family and friends, an endless stream of gifts, birthday parties, holiday get-togethers, camping trips, vacations to meet Mickey Mouse, his first Brewer game at County Stadium—you name it. Alex was so easy to love, and it showed. That little guy changed our lives forever, in the most incredible way.

Carrying Alex into the apartment for the first time felt surreal. The place was quiet, the crib already waiting, and it struck me how something so small could change the entire shape of our lives the moment he crossed the threshold. That first night at home, everything felt unusually still. I remember lying there listening for every sound, half afraid to fall asleep, knowing there was someone in the next room who depended on us completely. It was good to be home, but ultimately our time in the apartment with Alex was short. We soon packed up and moved back to Milwaukee, down the block from the very place where Christina and I had reconnected in 1993. Our first home was on 88th Street, just a half block south of Champion Chicken and the infamous Chicken Fest. I don't think we ever actually talked about it, but I was nostalgic knowing we lived so close to where our paths crossed again, setting us on this incredible life journey.

So much changed in those six years. College graduation, travel school, moving to and from another city, marriage, our first home, and the pinnacle of it all: having a child together. That's a lifetime for some people. But we've never been shy about figuring out what we want and going after it.

Later that night, I stood in the doorway of the nursery and looked at the crib I'd put together months earlier, finally understanding that the life I'd been imagining was now sleeping inside it.

CHAPTER 15: ...And Four, And Five

It seemed like the first two years of Alex's life flew by. Suddenly, the days were measured in nap schedules, diaper changes, and how quickly the next week seemed to arrive, but before we knew it, we were doing it all over again—only this time, we were a bit more prepared. Baby number two was on the way, and I think Alex may have been more excited than we were, if that's even possible. Just like the first time, we anxiously waited to find out what we were having, but one thing was for sure—Alex didn't care one way or the other. He just wanted a sibling to share his room with.

This ride to the hospital felt smoother than the first, and this baby was a lot more cooperative when it came to the actual delivery. I'm sure for Christina it wasn't any easier or less painful, but in typical fashion, she handled it all with grace and determination. I had it in my head that I was fully prepared to meet this baby—after all, I had already done this once before. I was wrong.

Once the baby decided it was time to arrive, it didn't waste any time—and just like that, she was here. She. It was a girl. I was overcome with emotion. I couldn't contain how excited I was to have a little girl. Olivia Madison was so beautiful—she looked like a little doll. She was so tiny compared to the active two-year-old I was used to carrying around that I was almost afraid to hold her. That didn't last long. All I wanted to do was hold that little princess. I knew right away: Olivia would be a Daddy's Girl, and I would love being a Girl Dad.

We should have seen it coming, but Olivia's arrival started the cycle all over again. She was now the star of the show—and why not? She was just so damn cute. She wasn't the first grandchild, but she was the first granddaughter. If we thought we had a lot of toys before, the onslaught of new, more girly items seemed to be delivered by the truckload.

Our tiny house was filling up, and before long, we made the move to a bigger space, back in Menomonee Falls. The kids could have their own rooms (even though they liked sharing), and we were in a good location for school to start in a couple of years.

Life was great. Alex was quickly developing into the quick-witted, smarty-pants that we all still know and love. Olivia spent her time keeping up with her brother while quietly blooming into a bright, compassionate soul all her own, and the two of them developed the close bond they still share today.

I'm guessing it didn't come as a surprise to Christina that I was going to drag my first-born son into the world of sports that I've always loved. Although I was a basketball nut, Alex really gravitated toward baseball, and we spent the next handful of years learning the intricacies of the game together. I mean, when he was asked what games he liked best at Chuck E. Cheese, he declared at the young age of four, *"I just really like baseball."* All that was left was for him to be a lefty—and well, that's exactly what happened.

And Olivia—I couldn't wait for her to be old enough to join dance. If I thought she was a doll before, when I saw her in her dance outfits, you could've put her on a shelf and sold her at a toy store. Did I mention that she was so damn cute? Now, had I known this dance thing would sign me up for a decade of making an ass of myself on stage—tripping over my two left feet—I might not have been as excited. But honestly, the adorable look on her face—the excitement she showed when she'd run out to meet me on that stage—it absolutely melted my heart. I wouldn't trade any of those awkward video moments for anything. I loved every minute of it.

We spent the first two years in our new home making the space our own and enjoying our young family. One of my favorite moments was painting the clubhouse with the kids, adding the Brewer logo to make it look like Bernie's Chalet, the Brewers' mascot's house. That thing was kind of falling apart, but at least it looked cool. The kids enjoyed the backyard, we added temporary pools from time to time, and Alex and I began what would become a lifelong activity—the little lefty pitching to me. I remember the game we'd play where he had to strike out three imaginary batters before walking in a run. If he did it successfully, he'd earn a pack of baseball cards. I didn't necessarily start his obsession with card collecting, but I absolutely added fuel to the fire.

A house, a boy, a girl—life was good. What could we be missing? Life with two kids had started to feel familiar, even comfortable, which is probably why what came next caught us so off guard.

Fast-forward a few years, there I was, lounging in our living room on the ugly plaid couch Christina had tricked me into buying, either half asleep or watching something on TV. I remember her walking down the hall and laying on the couch next to me. I figured she just wanted to be close, but after a minute or so, I noticed she was crying. After a quick mental scan to make sure I wasn't the source of those tears, I asked what was wrong. She sat up, turned around, looked me square in the eyes and said, *"I'm pregnant."*

It took a second to process, but I reached out, grabbed her, and gave her a big hug—to which she responded, *"You're not mad?"* To this day, I'm still not sure why she thought I would be upset. I must have made some off-hand comment about whether I wanted more kids, but I can honestly say I was just as excited to hear the news as I was the first two times. And since we already had a boy and a girl, I didn't even care what we were going to have. I was just excited to start that chapter again.

This time, temptation got the better of us, and we peeked in the envelope to find out the gender of the baby. I still can't believe we set up the crib and decorated it with boy décor, and my mom still didn't figure it out. Other than that, we did a pretty good job keeping it a secret.

Nine months later, our family was complete. Jacob Drew entered the world, and once again, I was beaming with pride. Alex and Olivia had a little brother to teach all their bad habits (just kidding), and we had another adorable little guy to smother with love.

Now, had I known this one was going to be a mini-me, I might have been even more excited from the get-go (if that's possible)—but who can predict something like that? I honestly don't know what we would have done without this final addition. Jacob was the last piece of the puzzle that is our amazing family. The five of us have had so many wonderful times together, and although people say no family is perfect, ours might be the exception to the rule. I found the most amazing girl to call my wife, and she gave me three incredible children to fill my heart. Without these four, my life would be empty.

Once again, we had outgrown our house, and just like we built our family, it was time to build our home. Selling the house our kids had grown up in and moving in with my in-laws temporarily was not an easy decision, but knowing what was at the finish line made it worthwhile. Two full years of living in our basement "apartment" was certainly challenging (and not really temporary), but honestly, I liked having our family of five so close together. And I know the kids really enjoyed being with their grandparents that whole time. Had they been older, it might not have worked, but at that point in our lives, it made a lot of sense.

It felt like an eternity, but when we finally moved into that house, for the first time in our married lives, it felt like we were truly home. Everyone had their own room, the kids had a big yard to play in, and even the unfinished basement (before it became a finished living space) provided a place for them to hang out. Cold nights sitting by the fire, a large kitchen to cook in, and enough garage space to finally park all our cars inside (and it was attached!). It was—and still is—a home I truly loved.

Life was cruising along, and our kids were hitting milestones. Alex moved quickly from one year of elementary school in our new town to middle school and then on to high school and college. Olivia followed right behind, chasing the same journey. And Jacob really experienced it all in that house— from 4K through high school. It's a home we never thought we'd leave, but life is never that predictable.

CHAPTER 16: XXX OOO

Not everyone gets lucky when it comes to in-laws. You hear the stories—awkward holidays, silent tensions, passive-aggressive comments over dinner. That was never my experience. From the very beginning, Tom and Patty welcomed me with open arms, a warm smile, and a quiet kind of trust that said, *"We're watching, but we're rooting for you."*

To be honest, I gave them a few reasons to raise an eyebrow in those early years. I was still figuring things out—young, a little rough around the edges, dating their daughter—their pride and joy. But even during those uncertain moments, there was never judgment or disapproval. Just patience. Steady support. And, maybe most importantly, belief. They believed in me, and in Christina's instincts. And they gave us space to become who we were meant to be.

Over time, that initial kindness evolved into something deeper. They weren't just Christina's parents anymore—they became an integral part of my life. When cancer entered the picture, and so much else fell apart, they became part of what held everything together. Quietly, steadily, without ever making it about themselves.

Tom is a classic example of a man who doesn't say much unless he really means it—but when he does speak, people listen. He's calm, even keeled, and more capable than he gives himself credit for. He can fix just about anything, and even if his methods are a little unorthodox at times, the job always gets done. He's a builder in more ways than one. After retiring, he spent countless hours in our basement, finishing it with skill and care—transforming it from a cold, empty space into something warm and livable. That wasn't just a favor. That was love.

Tom is not only handy, he's also incredibly generous with his time and talent—and patient enough to include me in his projects, which is saying something. I've never been the most capable when it comes to handyman work, but Tom never made me feel like that was a problem. He always saw it as an opportunity to teach, to include, and to connect.

While working on that basement, he would let me help whenever I wasn't busy with my full-time job. One particular weekend, we were installing the drop ceiling together. About halfway through, Tom realized we were short on supplies and needed to make a run to the hardware store. Before he left, he gave me a clear set of instructions for how to assemble the metal braces, and with the kind of hopeful trust you'd give to a slightly overconfident intern, he left me to it.

I lasted about five minutes before I ran into trouble. While trying to force one of the metal bars into place, it slipped and sliced open the palm of my hand. Bleeding and mildly panicked, I scrambled to clean it up and bandage myself up before Tom got back. I even managed to assemble a few pieces, so it didn't look like I'd completely fallen apart in his absence.

But I couldn't resist adding a little humor to the situation. I grabbed a scrap of paper and made a sign that read: *"Accident-Free Workplace: 0 Days."* When Tom came back and walked down the stairs, he looked around and saw the sign hanging proudly in the work area. *"What the heck happened?"* he asked, half-laughing already. When I held up my bandaged hand, we both cracked up. It's still one of my favorite memories of us working together—not because everything went smoothly, but because Tom always made me feel like I belonged in the process, even if I was bleeding from it.

And Patty—well, she's the heart of it all. She's got this beautiful way of loving people that's both generous and unspoken. She doesn't need the spotlight, and she certainly doesn't ask for thanks—but her love is felt in everything she does. Whether it's watching the kids, cooking a meal for the extended family, or simply being there with a hug at exactly the right time, she shows up.

That love extends deeply to her grandchildren, and they return it in kind. One of my favorite examples of this affection lives on Alex's arm. Every card Patty has ever given—to any of us, for any occasion—has ended the same way: *"XXX OOO."* It's her signature, her way of saying *"I love you"* without having to say it aloud. That little detail, so uniquely hers, left such an impression on Alex that he had it tattooed on his arm. Not because it looked cool, but because it meant something. Because it was a symbol of how deeply he feels her love.

Over the years, Christina and I have leaned on them more times than we can count. And not once—*not once*—have they ever made us feel like a burden. Their support has been constant. Their love, resolute. And even though our lives haven't been easy, Tom and Patty have never wavered in their commitment to our family.

When my own relationship with my parents broke down, they didn't try to replace anyone—but they quietly stepped into the space that was left behind. They offered the kind of safety and stability that I had lost. They showed me that "family" isn't just about biology. It's about presence. About love. About standing beside someone in the dark and staying there until the light comes back.

They've seen us through so much: new homes, new babies, surgeries, setbacks, milestones, meltdowns. Through it all, they've loved us the same—fiercely, generously, and without condition.

Patty has even said, more than once, that she considers me one of her own. Not just in words, but in the way she treats me. In the way she shows up. I didn't come from her, but I was welcomed by her. Loved by her. And that kind of love isn't something I take lightly.

So yes, I may have lost something in the fracture of my own family. But I gained something, too—something rare and priceless. I gained a second set of parents who became something even more profound than in-laws. They became my people. My foundation. My family.

And for that, I will always be grateful.

CHAPTER 17: My World

I've spent a significant amount of time, detailing most of the characters that make up my life story, but I'm going to spend a few moments honoring three of the lights that shine brightest in my world.

Dear Alex,

Or should I say, *"Scoop?"*

To say you changed our lives would be an understatement. From the moment you entered this world, you have brought Mom and I the kind of happiness that I can't truly describe. You were the first to push our journey from great to incredible, and I am so proud to call you, my son.

From the very beginning, you and I have shared something special. A connection that was easy, natural, and full of laughter. I remember looking at you as a baby—curious eyes, expressive face—and feeling that father-son spark that I didn't fully understand yet but knew was there. And over time, that spark became a fire.

Baseball has always been your thing. From the moment you stood in front of the TV, shouting *"Ball! Ball! Ball!"* at just a year old, it was clear that something about the game captured your heart. What I didn't realize then was how much it would also capture mine—not because I was suddenly obsessed with curveballs or pitch counts, but because baseball gave me a front-row seat to watch you become who you are.

Through the practices, the tournaments, the road trips, the games, good and bad—what I'll always remember isn't the stats. It's the time. It's the conversations between innings. The snacks on long car rides. The shoulder slumps after a rough outing and the grin when something finally clicked. I got to watch you chase a dream, and that gift is something I'll never take for granted.

I saw how hard you worked. I saw you lead, support your teammates, push through doubt and adversity. I watched a boy become a man on those mounds. But more than that, I saw the kind of human being you were becoming off the field—humble, loyal, quick-witted, kind.

There are moments that still play like highlights in my head: you being recognized at that tournament in Michigan, the all-star invite to Disney's Wide World of Sports, and of course, watching you toe the rubber for the Kenosha Kingfish. Simmons Field, packed with fans—kids chasing you down for autographs, the smell of brats in the air, your name over the loudspeaker. It was magic. Watching you in that jersey felt like watching a movie I never wanted to end.

I know the dream didn't end with a big-league contract, but honestly, you already won. You played the game you loved for as long as you could. You wore the uniforms, you walked out with your team, and you gave it everything you had. When you pitched your final game, your mom and I were prepared to console you—but instead, you were the one comforting us.

That says everything about who you are.

UW-Parkside gave you more than innings and memories—it gave you Hannah. You two have your own "how we met" story, one that might not start in grade school like your mom and me, but is no less rooted in love and shared joy. I still laugh thinking about her falling for you while you were dressed as a slutty police officer on Halloween. That's so you. Somehow ridiculous and charming all at once. And now, the two of you are married and beginning your own chapter. I'm so proud of the life you're building together. Oh, and we can't wait to meet your bundle of joy in July!

You've always been the comic relief in our family, but you're also our emotional core in so many ways. Your humor has gotten me through some of my hardest moments. You know just when to throw in a joke or hit a punchline that lightens the weight we're carrying. You have this rare gift of making things better just by being in the room.

Moving to Florida hasn't been easy—especially being so far from you. But every time we talk or spend time together, I'm reminded of how strong that bond is. You're not just my son, Alex. You're one of my best friends. I look at the man you've become—compassionate, hilarious, loving—and I couldn't be prouder.

Love you always,
Dad

Dear Olivia,

Liv. Boo. My little dancer. My partner in crime.

From the moment you came into our lives, you brought a

kind of joy that can't be explained—it can only be felt. You were so tiny, so delicate, and yet your presence was enormous. I remember being almost afraid to hold you at first because you looked like a porcelain doll. That didn't last long. I couldn't put you down. From the very beginning, you had me wrapped around your finger—and honestly, you still do.

Watching you grow up has been one of the greatest privileges of my life. Whether you were sneaking around to keep up with your big brother, spinning in those impossibly cute dance costumes, or swinging confidently in the front row of your volleyball games, you've always had this magical mix of poise and playfulness. I could see early on that you had your mom's grace, but your own kind of sparkle. And when you and I would practice for those daddy-daughter dances—I mean, how lucky was I to be the guy you wanted on that stage with you?

Now, let's be clear—I was *not* the most graceful partner. I've got two left feet, and those recital tapes prove it. But I would relive every clumsy spin, every awkward shuffle, and even that time I accidentally body-checked that poor little dancer next to us, just to see that look on your face when the crowd clapped and you knew we pulled it off together.

Beyond the dance floor, you've always been the one with the softest heart. You love your brothers with the kind of ferocious loyalty most people only dream of. You show up for people. You offer to help before anyone even asks. You have a kindness that sneaks up on you—not loud, not flashy, just *real* and consistent and deeply rooted in who you are. It reminds me of Kelly in so many ways.

You and I—we get each other. Whether it's trading ridiculous Instagram reels or daydreaming about house renovations we'll never actually do, we've got this rhythm. You share my taste for chaos in the kitchen and my addiction to gadgets we probably don't need. I love that about us. If we ever *did* click "buy now" on everything in our carts, our house would look like QVC and Amazon had a baby.

Liv, you're funny, thoughtful, strong, and deeply grounded. You're everything I hoped a daughter would be and so much more. I don't know how I got lucky enough to be your dad, but I count that blessing every single day.

So, go light up the world with that spark of yours. Just know that no matter how old you get, how far you go, or what you accomplish—I'll always see that little girl in a sparkly tutu, spinning around the living room, smiling up at me with all the love in the world.

Love always,
Dad

———————

Dear Jacob,
Jake. Bubbs. My mini-me.
From the very start, you've been the one who quietly stole my heart in ways I never saw coming. I don't know if it's because you're the youngest, or because you're my doppelgänger, or because we share the same third-child DNA—but watching you grow has been like looking in a mirror, one that somehow reflects both the past and the future at the same time.

You were always a little more reserved, a little more laid back than your older siblings—content to hang back, observe, figure things out in your own way, in your own time. And I saw that. I *recognized* that. Because I remember being that same kid, trying to carve out space in the shadows of louder voices. But just like me, you came into your own—gradually, confidently, and with a quiet strength that makes me incredibly proud.

You've got this natural calm to you. A steady hand. You don't demand attention, but when you speak, people listen. And when you lead, it's not about volume—it's about presence. I saw it when you played high school volleyball, stepping up on a team full of rookies, encouraging your teammates and showing a side of yourself that was ready to take the lead. I knew it before then, but that was a moment when I saw the man you were becoming.

And then there was *that* moment—the one I'll never forget. Standing in that gym, listening from a few feet away as you told Claire's parents why you were planning to choose the University of South Florida for college. You didn't know I was nearby. You weren't trying to impress anyone. You just said it: *"My dad's going to be getting treatment at Moffitt Cancer Center on USF's campus. That means I'll get to see him at least once a month. I want to be there for him."*

Jake… that moment cracked me wide open. Not because I needed you to be near me. But because you *wanted* to. Because you chose to build your life around love, around family, around being present. It said everything about your character—your loyalty, your heart, your strength. And I'll never, ever forget it.

We laugh about the hairline you've inherited (sorry, kid), but what I see when I look at you is someone better than I ever was at your age. Smarter, more compassionate, more centered. And every time I hear your voice—so deep now it still catches me off guard—I hear a young man with purpose.

I don't know exactly where your path will lead, but I do know this: whatever you decide to do, whatever you become, the world will be better for having you in it. You're already the kind of person people count on. The kind of son any parent would be lucky to have. And the kind of man I'm proud to stand beside—not just as your dad, but as your biggest fan.

So, take that big heart and that sharp mind and go make your mark. Just don't be surprised when I show up with a basketball, a bad dad joke, and some advice you didn't ask for.

With So Much Love,

Dad

––––––––––

We are blessed! Our children are amazing and have always made us proud. They have all experienced more on this earth than we really thought possible—some bad, but almost always good—some individually, but almost always together.

Likely a result of the how my family situation turned out, I've often lamented that you can't choose your family. Sure, you can choose your friends, your job and where you live, but your family is chosen for you. You can't control who your parents are or the siblings you'll share your life with, and in my case, it hasn't always been a fairy tale ending. But what I see in my kids, and how they truly love each other—it warms my heart to know they understand and appreciate how much that really means.

Enjoy them, world. They are the best!

CHAPTER 18: The Family You Find Along the Way

As much as our story is shaped by the family we were given, it's also defined by the people we choose to walk alongside us. Life has a way of introducing the right souls at the right time—people who don't share your blood but somehow understand you better than anyone else. After building a life with Christina and raising three amazing kids, we found ourselves surrounded by a few rare individuals who felt less like friends and more like family. And at the center of that chosen family are two people who have carried us through some of life's hardest and happiest moments.

As I said, you can't choose the family you are born into. And biologically, that's true. But if you're lucky—really lucky—you get to choose the people who walk beside you in life. The ones who hold space for you without needing to be asked. The ones who know your pain and meet you there with no judgment, just love. Some of the best conversations in our lives have happened on borrowed time—late nights after long days, weekend visits that ended too soon, and trips where the laughter started before we even unpacked. For Christina and me, those people are Tim and Karie.

Karie has been part of Christina's life for as long as she's been alive. They grew up together, attended St. Margaret Mary, and shared every milestone of childhood, adolescence, and early adulthood. Karie isn't just Christina's best friend—she's her chosen sister. And by extension, she became mine too.

When Christina and I began dating, Karie was always around. She wasn't a third wheel—she was part of the ride. So many of our early memories as a couple have Karie right there in the background, laughing with us, cheering us on, grounding us in friendship. And then, she met Tim.

They met early in college, and shortly after that connection, he enlisted in the United States Air Force. They got married not long after his basic training and began their journey of service, sacrifice, and family-building. Their first posting was in Destin, Florida—ironic, since we'd end up in Florida ourselves much later. After that, they settled in the Colorado Springs area, more than twenty years ago, raising their boys, Josh and Ryan, and building a life steeped in loyalty, grit, and grace.

There's always that lingering question when two best friends marry: *What if the husbands don't get along?* What if it's awkward or forced or just—not a fit? That fear disappeared the minute Tim and I met. In fact, somewhere along the way, we started joking that we might be even closer than the girls. And maybe we are—just don't tell them. I don't remember exactly what we talked about the first time Tim and I spent real time together—only that it never felt awkward, like we'd skipped the small talk and landed somewhere familiar right away.

Tim and I share a unique bond, forged not just through laughter, road trips and years of friendship, but through physical pain and emotional endurance. He spent 21 years in the United States Air Force, including multiple tours in the Middle East, and the wear and tear on his body from both service and genetics has been substantial. He's had surgeries, setbacks, and chronic discomfort—stuff that's hard to talk about with people who haven't lived it. But he and I? We talk about it. We get it. The frustration of wanting to feel *normal* again. The invisible weight that pain puts on your spirit. The silent toll it takes.

Then cancer came barreling into my life, and our friendship took on even deeper meaning. Of course, we had a huge support system—people who showed up with meals, prayers, texts, and rides. But Tim and Karie? They hold us up in ways that defy description. They know when to talk and when to just sit in the silence. They know when to distract us with joy and when to lean in with love. There have been long phone calls with Karie where we talk about how I can love Christina better, support her stronger, be more present through the chaos. There have been just as many calls with Tim where I check in on *him*, because he carries a weight too. There's a mutual respect, a true give and take that only happens between people who really, deeply love each other.

Karie has been an emotional lifeline for Christina and me alike. She somehow manages to know what we need before we do. Whether it's advice, encouragement, or just a well-timed laugh, she delivers. And Tim—well, my kids call him Uncle Tim, and that's not just a courtesy title. He *is* their uncle. In every meaningful sense of the word.

Uncle Tim is the guy you call when your car won't start, when your kid needs a pep talk, or when you just need a laugh. He says gift-giving is his love language, and he's not wrong. The man never shows up empty-handed. Sometimes I think he uses it as an excuse to visit the sporting goods store and buy a bunch of stuff he doesn't need—but we all benefit from that generosity, so who's complaining?

What makes this friendship so beautiful is how effortless it is. When we travel together—which we do as often as we can—it's like slipping into your favorite hoodie. Comfortable. Familiar. Filled with warmth and laughter. We've had dreams of one day living near each other again, of doing life side by side instead of across time zones. Maybe that day will come. Until then, we plan trips, carve out time, and stay close the way you do with people who matter.

The older I get—and the more uncertainty life throws our way—the more I realize how rare this kind of friendship is. People who see you completely, who accept your flaws, your fears, and your history. People who show up, even when it's inconvenient. Especially when it's inconvenient. People who laugh with you until your sides hurt and then sit quietly beside you when there's nothing left to say.

Tim and Karie aren't just our best friends. They are our chosen family. The kind of people you hope will be there at the end, because they've been there for everything that came before it.

If I've learned anything, it's this: blood may be thicker than water, but love—real love—is thicker than both. Even across miles and time zones, there's a comfort in knowing some people are never far from your life.

CHAPTER 19: Adversity Makes Us Stronger

Looking back now, it didn't feel like one diagnosis—it felt like a lineup. Three separate moments, spaced out just enough for us to catch our breath, but never long enough to feel safe. Christina's scare. Her surgery. And then mine. Each one arrived with its own fear, its own waiting, its own fallout. At the time, we treated them like isolated storms. Only later did I realize they were part of the same weather system.

Life isn't always the fairy tale that we hope and dream of. I vividly remember, very early in our marriage, when Christina discovered a lump in her breast and the subsequent anxiety we both felt, especially due to the history of breast cancer in her family. She unfortunately has too many warriors in her lineage who have dealt with this awful disease. I tried my hardest to be strong for her, but when she wasn't by my side, I let my guard down and was devastated, thinking about what could happen to her. Tests never seem to happen very quickly, but it truly felt like an eternity from the time Christina found the lump to when the doctors performed the mammogram to when they went in to do the lumpectomy. All the joy and incredible memories we had made to that point seemed so far away. I was determined to do whatever I could to get her through it, but at the same time, I felt so helpless. Why was this happening to her? Out of all the people in my life, she was the last person that deserved to go through something like this. Although I never told Christina, I was terrified that I would lose her. My mind raced back to the beginning of our relationship and those nine months when we weren't together, and I distinctly remembered how empty I felt inside. I wasn't going to let that happen again, especially by something that had no right to get in our way. At night, after Christina fell asleep, I'd sit alone at the kitchen table long after the lights were off, staring at the grain in the wood and wondering how much worse things could get.

Thankfully, everything was okay. The tumor was benign, and Christina had seemingly dodged a bullet—for now. After recovering from surgery, we felt like we had put that chapter safely behind us, and shortly thereafter, we began to build the family I just talked about. Life was back on track, all the way up to 2014, when cancer truly reared its ugly head. During another routine mammogram, images showed suspicious spots, this time much closer to the breast plate and much more difficult to examine. There we were, back to the tests and waiting game that no one wants to play.

We lived in a constant state of anticipation—jumping every time the phone rang, only to be told we'd have to wait a little longer. In the subsequent long days and weeks, we were not getting the answers we were desperate to hear. Eventually, we were sitting in a small exam room when the doctor finished explaining the options, the kind of quiet settling in that tells you something irreversible is about to be said. Ultimately, the best option in the doctor's opinion was to have a procedure to go in and biopsy the spots, and use that information to determine the next course of action. Faced with that as the "only viable option," what came next was, without a doubt, the bravest decision I have ever witnessed anyone make. When the doctor reiterated their plan as the best strategy moving forward, without hesitation, Christina asked if she could have a double-mastectomy and hopefully end the threat before it has a chance to get worse. I was blown away by her courage. To voluntarily put herself through grueling surgeries and alter the physical makeup of her body, without an instant of second thought—in that moment, I wished I had even a fraction of Christina's resolve. She truly is my hero.

It should be noted that Christina's intuition was correct and, following the removal of all breast tissue and the subsequent biopsies to determine exactly what we were dealing with, results showed that the spots were pre-cancerous, so removal was the right decision. Had the masses remained in there, they likely would have become cancer—Christina had beaten this awful disease to the punch.

What followed was a long road of additional surgeries, infections, expansion, and reconstruction that lasted well into 2015. Once again, I felt helpless, but I did all I could. I learned more about shampooing and conditioning hair than I ever thought a bald man could learn. Emptying surgical drains might be tough for some, but when it came to helping the love of my life, I was more than willing to do my part. Thankfully, she made it to the finish line and, although I thought it impossible, I see her stronger and more beautiful than I ever saw her before. Slowly but surely, our lives started to get back to *normal*. When everything finally slowed down, what stayed with me most wasn't the fear, but the quiet resolve we'd found together.

As I mentioned, I'm not the most overtly religious person. 13 years of parochial school, however, really ingrained in my head that nightly prayers are good for the soul. To this day, with very rare exceptions, I pray on a nightly basis. And if I wasn't someone who prayed before, I would have started anyway. I prayed and prayed, asking for Christina to be okay. What I didn't tell her until years later was that, as her surgery date drew near, I humbly asked God that, if cancer was His plan for our family, would He please give it to me instead. I obviously didn't want either of us to have to go through it, but if it had to be one of us, I wasn't going to let it be Christina. I'll never know for sure if the past ten years have been God answering my prayers, but in my heart, I want to believe it was.

CHAPTER 20: Prayers Answered

Our trip to Disney the following holiday season was special. Thanks to Alex's selection to an all-star team, we were able to escape the harsh Wisconsin winter and take the family down to the Florida sunshine. It was unseasonably hot that year, but balanced out by the refreshingly cool water of the pool at the rental house. It was just what we needed with the cloud of uncertainty hanging over our heads. Watching Alex play the game he loves, swimming in December and January, going to the theme parks with tens of thousands of other unexpectedly sweaty Disney enthusiasts, and just enjoying life with our family—it was the perfect trip. Shortly after we returned, I had the colonoscopy that would once again send our world into a flurry of worry and anxiety.

I don't remember that Friday very well. Whatever drugs they pumped me with erased my memory for the remainder of the day, but in talking about it with Christina afterwards, when the doctor briefed her following my procedure, she knew. I was blissfully unaware throughout the weekend, but deep down she already knew what I'd hear when the doctor reached out the following Monday.

When the call finally came, I stepped out and answered without really hearing much of what followed. I'm sure there was a greeting, maybe an introduction, but I only truly remember those three words nobody ever wants to hear: *"You have cancer."* I tried frantically to scribble down some instructions he was giving me, my hand shaking violently, as my heart sank into my stomach. Then the line went dead before I could think of what to say next. I stared at my phone for a second longer than necessary, then set it face down on the counter. Immediately, my thoughts wandered away from me and squarely on the four most important people in my life…Christina, Alex, Olivia, and Jacob. How was I going to share the news with them that had just been given to me? What does this all mean? Will I get a chance to at least see one of my children graduate from high school? All emotions and questions that have unfortunately been asked a million times by far too many people.

I wanted to tell Christina in person, but I couldn't hold all these emotions in for the half-hour drive home. Eventually, I stepped into an empty conference room and made the hardest call I've ever made in my life. She answered the phone, and when she heard my shaky voice, I think she already knew what I was going to say. I don't cry often (well, I didn't, but that has all changed), but in that moment, we cried together as we tried to process how our lives would change forever. All I wanted to do was reach through the phone and give Christina a huge hug and let her know that I was going to be okay—something I wasn't sure of at that point, but words that would hopefully comfort her somewhat. It was a long ride home, but when I finally walked through the door, we shared that hug that I wish I could have delivered earlier.

We decided it would be best to wait until we had more information before we broke the news to the kids, and after weeks of tests and scans, I had an official diagnosis—Stage III colorectal cancer. A long battle was staring me in the face, but I felt confident that I would win the fight. I mean, I had just watched Christina navigate through a similar situation with such grace and courage, and the example she set for me two years earlier is the only reason that I had the strength to fight. Unfortunately, now it was time to tell our young children that, after having watched their mother struggle through a difficult battle, it was Dad's turn to do the same thing.

We sat the kids down together in the living room, close enough that we didn't have to raise our voices. We kept the details simple—just the truth they needed, no more. Enough to be honest, but not so much that it took away their sense of safety. We wanted them to leave that conversation knowing one thing above all else: that their dad was going to fight, and that we believed he was going to be okay.

That was, hands down, the toughest conversation we'd ever had with our children, but to their credit, they processed the news about as well as you could expect a 16-, 14-, and 10-year-old to, given the information they were hearing. Yes, there were a lot of emotions, but the way we explained it and instilled a sense of positivity was exactly how they needed to hear the news.

Before going to bed, I checked on each of them, watching them sleep, needing to see with my own eyes that they were okay.

That year sucked, but I did my best to tackle every milestone with a smile on my face. Some days, that smile didn't make it past the driveway—I'd sit in the car for a few extra minutes, hands on the wheel, just gathering enough energy to walk inside. I said it often throughout 2016 and a lot since, that mental health is just as important as physical health. On the days it felt hardest, I'd retreat to the bedroom in the middle of the afternoon and lie fully dressed on top of the covers, phone face down beside me, listening to the house breathe—reminding myself that if I didn't remain positive throughout the journey, there was no way I'd make it to the finish line. I knew that would be tough, but I had to do it—not just for me but for Christina and the kids. She made it a lot easier to do so. The love and support that she showered me with that year was nothing short of incredible. I know, deep down, she was struggling emotionally, but she rarely showed it to me. I know for a fact that I wouldn't have made it to the end without her, and for that I am forever grateful. Christina really did save my life!

Getting to the end has never really felt like the finish line, since the lasting effects of that year have not subsided, but in the months leading up to my 5-year cure date, it finally started to feel like we could get back to where we were before our battles. In my head, I had earmarked June 21, 2021, as the date that would allow us to put it all in our rearview mirror and get back to *normal*.

I was anxious for that day to get here and felt like it would have been a restart of sorts...almost like hanging a new calendar on the wall, but instead of January 1st being the first day, it would have June 21, 2021, as the first day of the rest of our lives. I thought it would be "just another day" that I would quietly celebrate in my head, but as you can imagine, my emotions really got the best of me. I couldn't explain it, but I sat on the guest bed at the house of our best friends, Tim and Karie, in Colorado, crying for quite a bit of time. Christina checked on me and found me sobbing, and like she has always done, wrapped her arms around me and held me close. She asked me why I was sad, and I told her that I wasn't—these were tears of joy and, deep down, I believed they were. Once again, she was there to pick me up.

CHAPTER 21: The Ones Who Walk with You

I started my professional career, after graduating from the University of Wisconsin, with a dream of working in sports. During my five years in Madison, I had the great fortune of working with the Badger Basketball team. I love basketball, and it was the perfect job for me. It may have hindered my studies a bit (okay, I definitely spent more time in the gym than in the classroom), but I loved every minute of it—practices, games, travel to away venues. It was the best. And the lifelong friendships I made with players, coaches, and fellow managers are a blessing I'll never take for granted. That "job" had me believing I would spend my life dedicated to the world of sports.

Shortly after graduation, I began a seasonal position in season ticket sales with the Milwaukee Brewers. Realizing quickly that I am the world's worst salesman, I shifted into a role in ticket operations, which—after three seasons—became the springboard to my full-time gig at the Greater Milwaukee Open, a PGA Tour event in town. Once again, my tenure would only last three years, but this time, I moved away from the dream.

A job in sports was not in my long-term future, so I shifted my focus. Kelly's best friend, and really another "big sister" to me, was Ami B. I had known her my whole life. She spent the better part of her youth at our house, and she always looked out for me like a big sister would. Ami worked at a marketing agency—but not just any agency. GMR Marketing distinguished itself by building physical experiences on behalf of brands and taking those experiences to moments of passion for consumers, like concerts and sporting events. It always sounded incredible to me, and when the opportunity presented itself, I asked if GMR was hiring. Long story short, Ami was the conduit into the career I've had ever since. Twenty-two years (and counting) later, I'm still there and still loving the experience. I've seen and done so many unbelievable things in my time at GMR, and I feel blessed to be a part of the journey.

Unfortunately, Ami left the agency shortly after I started, so we never really got to enjoy our time as co-workers. Still, she had already set my course in motion, and I'd soon find another incredible person waiting in the next chapter.

Experiences are one thing, but what I'll forever be grateful for are the friendships. I've often said, *"I'm never the smartest person in the room, but I've been successful by simply building relationships."* I'm a people person, and that instinct has carried me throughout my career. Many of my closest friends are current and former colleagues—all of whom transitioned to a de facto support system over the past decade. There are too many cheerleaders in my corner to name them all individually, but they know who they are and how much I appreciate them.

There is one person, however, who has always been there for me—even before all of this cancer bullshit. She's been a colleague, a boss (at times), a mentor—but most importantly, a best friend.

Elke is one of the few people at GMR who can say she's been there longer than me. When I say I'm never the smartest person in the room, Elke is the opposite of that. She is brilliant—and it shows. She's universally loved and a true friend to everyone we work with.

I met Elke a couple years before we started working together. She likely doesn't remember, but it was a group gathering at a bar in Milwaukee, and due to my connection with Ami, we happened to be in the same place at the same time. I don't recall much—probably a simple introduction and an exchange of pleasantries. But when we began working together a few years later, our connection was instant. We share the same interests, the same humor, the same appreciation for Chris Cornell as a lyrical genius—and so much more.

We also share something else. Elke is a cancer survivor and someone who still battles to this day. For privacy reasons, I won't go into more detail, but I mention it to give context. Elke is someone who truly understands. It helps to have a best friend I can confide in, complain to, ask questions of, cry with, laugh with—and just exist with.

So, let's go back to 2016. That fateful call from my doctor. The excruciating wait to get home and hug Christina. All the thoughts racing through my head as I sat in the office, processing the news. I felt like I was on an island. I wasn't prepared to share this with anyone—not until I had a chance to tell my wife and family—but at the same time, I just needed something. Someone. I felt empty. My world had turned upside down.

I'd been answering emails and nodding through meetings all morning, but by then my chest felt tight and my hands wouldn't stop shaking. Where do you go when you instantly feel like all hope is lost? For me, the answer was simple.

I stood outside the window to her office, trying to see if she was available, tears welling up in my eyes. Elke knew. She dropped what she was doing and waved me in. I struggled to get the words out between sobs, but I didn't even have to. Again, Elke knew. She leapt out of her chair, raced over, and gave me exactly what I needed: a huge hug. We stood there for what seemed like forever, and for the first time since the call, I felt safe.

We spent the next hour just talking. She, of course, told me that—whatever I needed—she was there for me. I already knew that, but the words were comforting. She helped me figure out the best way to tell Christina and reminded me that, in this moment, nothing else matters but my family. She encouraged me to make that call to my wife, and then she sent me home.

I didn't know it at the time, but this cancer bond would be forever. Neither of us will ever truly be cancer-free, but we're both seemingly at peace with that. We're able to connect and talk on a level that, unless you've had the misfortune of going through something like this, you wouldn't understand.

Elke has been a rock emotionally; she's also my support behind the scenes. She's always checking on me. When the race to the finish line between me and cancer seems to be tilting in favor of the disease, she is always quick to spring into action. With the support of so many wonderful people at my agency, Elke makes sure that—with everything going on in my life outside of the office—work is never one more reason to feel stressed or overwhelmed. It may sound simple, but that gift is a tremendous weight off my shoulders.

I'm getting ahead of myself a bit, but as recently as February of 2025, Elke and I were on a work trip to Arizona. We carpooled to an evening event, just the two of us, and it gave us time to talk. I mean, we've always talked, but this time, the conversation was deeper than it had ever been before. We talked about our families and our future. We talked about the lives we've lived and how this job has given us so much. We talked about the end—an idea that once terrified me but now feels more like a reality we've both come to terms with. We walked in circles once we parked. We talked some more. We laughed. We cried. We hugged.

I wish, for everyone reading this book, that you could have the opportunity to meet Elke, even for just a few moments. Your life would change—mine has. She's just that type of person. She gives so much and asks for nothing in return. There aren't a lot of people in this world like Elke, and I'm blessed to call her one of my best friends.

I should mention that Ami—the rope that strung so many of us together, and the knot that keeps us tethered—was also a cancer warrior. You can surmise by the past-tense being used here, that Ami has moved on to become a cancer angel. She received her Stage IV diagnosis at the age of 40, battled like hell for almost a decade, but unfortunately succumbed to this awful disease a few years ago. The greatest rockstar to never take the stage…Stay Gold, Ami B.

INTERLUDE: A Shocking Mistake

When I first started chemo, one of the earliest warnings I got was about neuropathy. Numbness and buzzing in my feet, fingertips and the edges of my ears. It all sounded like fine print—until it wasn't. The tingling never left my feet, and there were weeks when I couldn't feel the difference between holding a pen or a paperclip. But the weirdest side effect? My throat.

For six months, I couldn't drink anything colder than room temperature water. Not because it gave me a headache or made me shiver—but because it felt like swallowing an electric fence.

One day, not long after my first official round of chemo, I came home still tethered to the pump that would administer more of the drug over the next 48 hours. We were prepping for a road trip to Minnesota—Alex had a college baseball showcase, and I was determined to be there, cancer or not.

It was warm outside. I was sweating and tired and instinctively grabbed an ice-cold Gatorade from the back of the car.

Big mistake.

The second that liquid touched my throat, I spit it out— immediately and violently—straight across the back of the SUV. It felt like someone had stuck a taser in my esophagus and cranked it to full power. I doubled over, half coughing, half laughing, while Christina looked at me like I'd just been struck by lightning.

It was hilarious. Painful, yes—but hilarious. The kids couldn't stop laughing, and once I recovered, neither could I. It was one of those absurd moments you just had to experience to understand. Lesson learned: room temperature only.

Cancer taught me a lot. One of the most important lessons? Always read the fine print—and never underestimate a Gatorade in August.

CHAPTER 22: The Next Chapter

At the time, it felt like an emotional release in Colorado—just a moment on a bed, alone with my thoughts—but I see now it may have been something more. In hindsight, I wonder if my body knew what was going on and those bedside tears in Colorado were a precursor to the news we received one month later. Shortly after starting this new journey, and looking back, the signs were beginning to present themselves. The loss of appetite, the weight loss, the extreme fatigue. I know we had a busy month leading up to that fateful CT scan, but these symptoms were more pronounced than they've ever been for me. As I write this, we're still holding out hope that we'll get good news someday, but I want everyone to know that no matter how intensely this battle rages, I will fight with everything in me to beat it once again.

Almost five years into this new clash, dealing with cancer on a daily basis, my mind always goes back to Christina and the kids. During the worst stretches, I sometimes stop moving through the day and start hiding from it—sitting on the edge of the bed, shoes still on, not ready to rejoin whatever comes next for my family. I can handle whatever this disease wants to do to my body, but what I can't stand is the thought of what it will do to the four most important people in my life. If I didn't have them, I'm not sure how much fight I'd have left in me. But the thought of not being here for them, the most important people in my life, not being able to experience all the wonderful milestones that our children have in front of them and not being able to live out this dream of fully experiencing our new life in Florida—it breaks my heart. The thought of all the pain that they will have to endure is crushing me inside, but it also provides me with the motivation, once again, to fight like hell and be there for all the wonderful moments to come.

Someday, we'll be able to look back and appreciate all that we've gone through and clearly see the positives that came out of all this. That sounds weird to say, but we've been blessed with so much to this point, and these struggles have only made us stronger. I'd like to think that I've been a good husband all these years, but looking back on it, I certainly could have been better. I went through a period where, emotionally, I wasn't always there for Christina…I almost took her for granted. She has always loved me unconditionally and I haven't always shown that same level of affection in return. For that, I am truly sorry! But, like I said, watching her fight her battle and then having to go through it myself, it reminded me how much I really have and that I should show Christina the love and affection that she deserves. If it's possible, I love her more now than I ever have before, and I feel blessed to know that our struggles are what opened my eyes to that.

And our children—what can I say except that they will be some of the strongest human beings on the face of the earth. If I thought I was heart-broken the first two times we had to sit down with them and break the news, this last time was exponentially tougher. They were older, and they understood everything better. They watched us both struggle through our battles, and it must have been excruciating for them. To have to do that all over again is not fair, and I feel awful that I'll be the source of their anguish once again, this time, without a positive finish line. But, like I said, they are amazing kids, and they will be there with us, fighting just as hard. You know, there are a lot of parents who claim their kids are the best in the world, but we're the only ones who can say that and know it's true. We couldn't have asked for more perfect, loving, and exceptional children, and the world is certainly a better place with them in it. We did that! If there's any gift or lasting legacy we can give this world, it's those three amazing human beings. Alex, Olivia, and Jacob…I love them more than life itself!

Whatever comes next, the one thing that hasn't changed—and never will—is how intensely I love my family.

INTERLUDE: Cancer In the Middle

Cancer is often described as a personal journey.

And in the most literal sense, it is. It happens inside one body. One set of scans. One chart with your name on it.

But that's never been the whole truth for us.

Cancer doesn't stay contained. It spreads outward—into waiting rooms, kitchens, car rides home. Into conversations that start with *"we need to talk"* and never quite return to *normal*. It settles in the middle of a family and changes how everyone stands, how everyone breathes.

Christina has lived this disease alongside me, not as a bystander, but as a constant. She shows up. Every time. She waits. Every time. And every time they call my name, she lets go—just enough—to keep moving forward. That space she occupies, between strength and breaking, is where so much of this story actually lives.

The kids grew up there too.

Not in a single moment, not because of one conversation— but because uncertainty became familiar. Because worry arrived early. Because resilience wasn't optional. They learned, without choosing to, how to live with answers that change and futures that don't stay fixed. And still, somehow, they learned how to laugh. That might be the bravest thing of all.

Cancer has a way of inserting itself into the pauses. The space between scans. The space between relief and fear. The space between "we're okay" and "what if we're not."

That's where we live now. In the middle.

We don't measure time the same way anymore. We don't stockpile certainty. We don't pretend tomorrow is promised. The small stuff fell away somewhere along the line—not because it didn't matter, but because something else mattered more.

Moments.

Hands held a little longer. *"I love you"* said without hesitation. Ordinary days that feel quietly extraordinary just because they exist.

Cancer has taken plenty from us. That's undeniable. But it's also clarified things with a brutal kind of honesty.

What matters.

Who matters.

What's worth fighting for.

This isn't a story about surviving alone. It never was.

It's about what happens when a family learns to stand together in the middle—not knowing what comes next, but choosing, every day, to keep showing up anyway.

INTERLUDE: Close Enough To Carry It

Standing together didn't always mean standing alone.

Some of the weight cancer brought into our lives stayed with our family. But some of it was quietly shared—lifted by people who were close enough to notice the strain before we ever had to name it.

That kind of support doesn't announce itself. It doesn't come with grand gestures or perfect words. Sometimes, it simply lives nearby.

Christina's sister, Lisa, and her husband, Jon, built their home right next door to ours, but what they really built was a shared life. Our kids didn't grow up as cousins—they grew up as siblings. Backyards blended together. Doors stayed open. The line between "their house" and "our house" never felt all that important.

When cancer entered our lives, that closeness mattered in ways I didn't fully understand at the time.

Lisa became part of the inner circle without hesitation. During surgeries and procedures, when Christina was sitting in waiting rooms, staring anxiously at the clock, waiting for a doctor to appear with news, Lisa was on the short list of people receiving updates—sometimes minute by minute. Not because anyone asked her to be, but because she was already there. Already invested. Already steady. That kind of presence doesn't need recognition. It just shows up and stays.

Jon carried things quietly too. He never needed to say much. He just made sure we knew we weren't alone—whether that meant stepping in with the kids, handling something that didn't need to become another burden, or simply being nearby when the weight felt heavy.

Their kids were part of the rhythm of our home in the most natural way. Ordinary days mixed with hard ones. Laughter coexisted with worry. Life didn't stop just because things were difficult, and somehow that helped all of us keep going.

And then there's Ryan.

Ryan is their oldest child but has always felt like another son to me. That bond didn't come from intention or effort—it just existed. He talks to me about everything. The big moments. The small ones. The things that feel too complicated or heavy to bring anywhere else. Sometimes it's easier for him to lean on me than even his own parents, and I've never taken that lightly.

When I had to tell him about the cancer the second time, his reaction cut deeper than I expected. His emotions were immediate and intense. In that moment, he wasn't processing diagnoses or statistics. He was grieving the idea that he might be losing his uncle—someone he saw as another father. That kind of love leaves a mark. On both of us.

Having them next door didn't make cancer easier. It didn't soften the diagnoses or shorten the recovery. But it changed how we carried it. It meant support didn't require planning. It meant help was close enough to feel instinctive. It meant none of us had to face the hardest moments in isolation.

Families are built in many ways. Some by blood. Some by choice. Some by proximity that turns into something much deeper over time.

The house next door was never just a house.

It was part of our foundation.

CHAPTER 23: The End Is the Beginning

So let me go back to our beginning—those brief moments at the gas station. Who would have thought that her dad's habit of buying used cars that weren't always the most reliable would end up being the universe's way of putting us on the same path. One small inconvenience. One ordinary moment. And somehow, everything changed.

When I look at Christina every morning, I still see that same girl who lit up my world. The girl I just wanted to talk to, even if only for a minute. Time hasn't erased that—it's refined it. It's layered it with history, with shared pain and shared joy, with a life we didn't plan but chose again and again.

To have the chance to spend nearly my entire life with her is more than I ever dreamed possible. She is the greatest thing that has ever happened to me. That hasn't changed. If anything, it's only become clearer. I still tell her every morning, *"I love you more today,"* and I mean it—because after everything we've been through, love isn't static. It grows. It deepens. It earns weight.

I don't know what the future holds. I don't know how many mornings we get, or how many chapters remain. But I do know this: Christina has walked every hard road beside me without hesitation. She became things she never signed up to be—caregiver, advocate, steady presence—while never letting go of who she already was.

Someday, as the years go by and we sit next to our pool in Florida, I hope we'll look back and smile—not because it was easy, but because it was ours. The good memories will rise naturally, and the harder ones will soften around the edges. We'll know that every turn we took, every moment we endured, mattered.

People say there's no such thing as a perfect couple. Maybe they're right—if perfect means untouched or effortless. But if perfect means choosing each other through uncertainty, through fear, through joy, and through everything in between, then I believe we are exactly that.

Christina—I love you more than you could ever imagine. Thank you for everything you've done for me and for our kids. The end of this chapter doesn't feel like an ending at all. It feels like the beginning of whatever comes next.

And whatever that is, I'm grateful it's with you.

. . .

In My Chosen Life, survival required redefining what "normal" meant — not as comfort, but as constancy. We found our footing in the middle of the storm by holding onto each other and making peace with the unknown.

III

Reflections

CHAPTER 24: Things I Learned Too Late

Some lessons arrive like a gentle whisper. Others hit like a brick to the chest. The most profound truths in my life didn't come in the classroom or through books. They came in the silence of hospital rooms, in the moments between scans, in the cracks between ambition and exhaustion.

I've spent a good chunk of my life trying to get it "right." Be a good man. A good husband. A great dad. And somewhere in that pursuit, I bought into a lie—one that's spoon-fed to people like me from an early age. That working harder, pushing more, sacrificing yourself for your career, your family, your future— would eventually pay off.

But here's the truth: I pushed too hard.

I worked through symptoms I shouldn't have ignored. I silenced pain that needed a voice. I believed that showing up to everything, never missing a beat, never complaining, never needing rest—made me strong. It made me dependable. And it also made me sick.

By the time I admitted something was wrong, it was well past the point of early warning signs. I look back now and think: *"What if I had said something sooner?"* What if I had raised my hand at work, or at home, and admitted that I was drowning beneath the surface of "fine"?

But the world rewards people who grind, not those who rest. It pats us on the back for our stamina, not our self-awareness. And so, I kept going. I wore my stress like a badge of honor, thinking I was setting an example. Maybe I was. But not the one I hoped to be.

Here's what I learned too late: strength doesn't mean doing it all. Strength is knowing when to stop. When to ask for help. When to say, *"This isn't normal, and I'm scared."*

I also learned that perfection is a myth—and the pursuit of it is a slow form of self-destruction. I wasted time worrying about being the perfect parent, the ideal partner, the model employee. And in that pursuit, I sometimes missed the moments right in front of me. I should have sat longer at the dinner table. I should have taken more sick days. I should have said yes to more games of catch, even when I was tired. I should have spoken up—about my pain, my fears, my needs.

Another hard truth: people won't always give you permission to slow down. You must give it to yourself. And if you wait until you're "allowed" to take care of yourself, it might already be too late.

I also learned, far too late, how fast time passes. Not just the cliché of how quickly kids grow up—but how quickly it can all change. One phone call, one test result, one sharp pain in your side—and the story you thought you were writing turns into a completely different book.

I regret some things, of course. But mostly, I just wish I had learned earlier to live from a place of presence instead of performance. To sit in stillness, not just accomplishment. To be okay with being still enough to feel, rather than constantly moving to avoid feeling too much.

But the silver lining in learning these truths late is that—I *did* learn them. And with the time I have now, I am doing things differently. I'm more honest. More open. I say *"no"* to the things that steal my energy and *"yes"* to what fills my cup. I speak up when something hurts. I let people in, even when it's uncomfortable. I rest. I listen. I love more gently.

So maybe this isn't a list of regrets. Maybe it's a roadmap—written backwards—for someone else to follow sooner than I did.

If you're reading this and you're pushing too hard, ignoring the pain, pretending everything's fine when it isn't—pause. Take a breath. Tell someone. Go to the doctor. Take the day off. Let your body speak. Let your loved ones in. Don't wait for the crash. Trust me—I've already learned that lesson for you.

CHAPTER 25: What I Leave Behind

If you ask most people what they want to leave behind, they'll probably say something big. A company. A name. A fortune. A story worth repeating.

But me? I just want to be remembered as a good man who loved his family more than anything else.

I've lived a complicated life—marked by diagnoses, loss, and pain—but none of that is the headline. The real story is about the people I got to share it with. It's about Christina. About Alex, Olivia, and Jacob. About Kelly. About Andrew. Even Adam, in his own way. And yes, it's about my parents, too— flawed as they were, they shaped me.

It's also about the moments that never made the highlight reel but mattered the most. Sitting on the floor building Legos. Playing old man softball on Thursday nights. Holding hands during chemo. Whispering *I love you* one last time to my dad, even if he didn't get to hear it.

I've made peace with a lot—more than I thought I ever would. I've faced my mortality, my grief, my guilt, and even the parts of myself I wasn't proud of. I've been forgiven. I've forgiven. And more importantly, I've learned to let go of what I can't carry anymore.

Some days, I still feel like that kid in Milwaukee—sharing a tiny bedroom with my brothers, watching my sister become a force of nature, trying to make sense of a world that felt both safe and wildly unfair. Other days, I feel like a 51-year-old father of three, just trying to hold on to every single moment because I know how quickly it all goes.

Christina once said that everything we've been through has made us stronger. I think she's right. The hardest parts of our life together are what bound us the tightest. And in some strange, cosmic way, cancer didn't break us—it revealed us. It peeled back everything unimportant until all that was left was what mattered most.

This memoir isn't a farewell letter. It's a thank-you note—to everyone who's been a part of my life. To those who loved me, even when I wasn't easy to love. To those who challenged me. To those who taught me something. And especially to those who stood by me.

Florida, for us, has become more than a destination. It's a symbol. Of healing. Of sunshine after the storm. Of soaking in joy while we can. It's where we've planted our new roots, and where I hope Christina and the kids can continue to grow, even when I'm no longer around to water the soil.

If you take anything from this book, let it be this: life doesn't have to be perfect to be beautiful. And *normal*? It's a myth. We all carry something—scars, secrets, struggles. What matters is how we love through it.

So, love big. Laugh often. Apologize when you need to. Let go of what weighs you down. And when in doubt, choose your family.

Because in the end, that's what we leave behind.

CHAPTER 26: The Thief and the Teacher

Cancer is a thief. It steals the things you don't realize you've come to depend on—not all at once, but slowly, methodically. It takes your time, your energy, your routines. It robs you of the ability to assume that tomorrow will look like today, and it forces you into a world where everything is uncertain. And yet, it also has a strange way of giving back. Not because it's generous, but because when you lose enough, what remains is often something rare and valuable.

I'll start with what it took.

It took my sense of physical invincibility. Not that I was ever delusional—I wasn't doing Ironman competitions or benching 300 pounds. But I was able. I was steady. I could wake up, go to work, coach a game, mow the lawn, chase the kids. I could lift groceries without flinching. I could carry the burden of life without having to think about how heavy it had become. When cancer showed up, all that changed. There were days when I couldn't get out of bed. Moments when I had to think twice before standing up. Seasons of life when I moved more slowly than a man my age should.

It took time. Countless hours in waiting rooms. Entire days lost to infusions, scans, and procedures. Milestones spent sitting under fluorescent lights while a machine pumped chemicals through my body. I missed events. I rescheduled plans. I sat out on things I used to take for granted—dinner with friends, trips with family, even just going to a movie or out for coffee. Time, it turns out, is the most precious currency we have. And cancer is greedy.

It took control. My calendar used to be mine. My body used to listen to me. Now, I answer to scans and appointments and treatments. I answer to doctors and blood counts and fatigue levels. I'm no longer the one behind the wheel—cancer took that too.

It took pride. There's a certain vulnerability in being seen at your weakest. In having to ask for help to walk across a room. In being too tired to play with your kids or too nauseated to enjoy a meal. You start to feel less like yourself and more like a shell of the person you used to be. I hated that part. Still do, if I'm honest.

But that's not the whole story.

Because cancer, as cruel as it is, also gave me things I never expected.

It gave me perspective. The kind that only comes when everything is stripped away and you're forced to confront what actually matters. Spoiler alert: it's not work emails or home improvement projects or social media likes. It's the people who sit with you when you're at your worst. It's the kid who hugs you extra tight before school. It's a quiet walk around the block or a night on the couch with the person you love. Perspective is one hell of a gift.

It gave me presence. I used to live in the next moment—planning, preparing, checking the boxes. Cancer made me slow down. Made me pay attention. Made me savor the little things: a funny text from Alex, Olivia baking in the kitchen, Jacob sitting next to me watching the Bucks. I stopped living in the someday and started appreciating the now.

It gave me connection. There's a vulnerability in illness that breaks down walls. I've had conversations I never would have had otherwise. I've been loved in ways I never expected. Friends became family. Coworkers became lifelines. Strangers became sources of inspiration. The humanity that showed up for me—in texts, in meals, in moments—reminded me that I'm not alone in this.

It gave me clarity. I used to say *"yes"* to things because I thought I should. Because I didn't want to let people down. Now? I say *"yes"* because I want to. And I say *"no,"* too. Without guilt. Cancer taught me that boundaries aren't selfish—they're survival.

It gave me the chance to model something real for my kids. Not perfection. Not superhuman strength. But honesty. Resilience. A willingness to keep showing up, even when things are hard. I don't want them to remember me as the dad who had cancer. I want them to remember that I kept trying. That I laughed when I could. That I let them see the hard stuff. That I never stopped loving them with everything I had left.

And it gave me Christina. Not in the literal sense—she was mine long before this fight—but in the truest, most tested version of the word. There is no hiding in marriage when cancer enters the picture. There is only rawness. Realness. She has seen me broken, worn out, scared, angry, hopeful, numb. She's been there for all of it. And somehow, she still smiles at me like I'm worth sticking around for. That kind of love—that daily choosing—it's not something you can fake.

Cancer didn't create that, but it sure as hell confirmed it.

So yes, cancer took a lot.

But it also stripped away the noise, leaving only what truly matters. And for that—not the pain or the loss, but the clarity— I am, in some odd way, grateful.

CHAPTER 27: Courage to Heal

There's a strange stigma around therapy—like it's only for people who are "broken," or for those who've completely fallen apart. For a long time, I believed some version of that lie myself. I thought needing help meant I had failed—that I wasn't strong enough to deal with life on my own. But here's what I've learned: *strong* people ask for help. Strong people *seek out* ways to get better. And therapy isn't weakness—it's one of the most courageous things you can do.

We don't hesitate to call a mechanic when the car breaks down or go to a dentist when a tooth aches. But when the pain is emotional—when the thoughts are too heavy, or the sadness doesn't lift—too many of us try to tough it out in silence. I hope that, if you see anything in my story that feels familiar—if you've ever felt numb, overwhelmed, exhausted, stuck—you'll give yourself the same permission I did: the permission to talk to someone. To open up. To heal.

Cancer changed my body. Therapy changed my mind.

I've always believed in staying strong—for my wife, for my kids, for myself. But after the dust settled from my first diagnosis, and I was technically "in the clear," something inside me didn't feel like it had healed. I told everyone I was okay. I tried to believe it myself. But the truth was, I didn't feel well physically and wasn't happy. I wasn't even sure I remembered what happiness felt like.

That's when I sought therapy for the first time.

I had never done that before—not seriously. But I'd hit a wall mentally, and I knew that if I didn't deal with the weight I was carrying, it would crush me. So, I found a therapist who works specifically with cancer patients. A good one. And we started talking.

One of the most pivotal moments of that first round of counseling came when I tried to explain what I was feeling. I told my therapist that I wasn't depressed in the classic sense—I wasn't hopeless or numb—but I also wasn't joyful. I felt like I was simply existing. And existing looked like eating meals without tasting them and watching days blur together because nothing felt worth anticipating. Just going through the motions. And then I said something that surprised even me:

"I don't want to just exist. I want to live."

That hit hard. I remember saying it and immediately tearing up. Because I knew it was true. I wasn't living. Not really. I was surviving winter after winter in Wisconsin—hibernating through the cold months, stuck in a place that didn't allow me to fully experience life year-round. I needed something more. Something different. Something *new*.

That's when the seed was planted to move to Florida.

It wasn't a rash decision. It was the result of months of processing, journaling, talking. But therapy gave me permission to imagine a different life—a *better* life. It was in that room, during those sessions, that the idea of moving to Florida stopped being a fantasy and became a lifeline. Therapy didn't give me the answers. It permitted me to dream a different version of my life—one that wasn't just about surviving, but about actually being *alive*. And eventually, I made that dream real.

But the work didn't stop there.

After my second diagnosis, the toll was heavier. Physically, I was declining. Mentally, I was unraveling. My care team— people I trust deeply—urged me to go back to therapy. This time, it was about more than location or seasons. It was about purpose.

In one session, I found myself spiraling into a feeling of uselessness. I told my therapist that I felt like my time to "change the world" had passed. That the window had closed. That, maybe, the best I could hope for now was just to fade quietly.

And then she looked at me and asked a simple question that I'll never forget:

*"Why do you need to change **the** world? Why can't you just focus on changing **your** world?"*

That question flipped a switch in me.

I had spent so much time focused on what I couldn't do anymore, I forgot to see what I *was* doing. Loving my family. Writing this book. Having hard conversations. Laughing. Crying. Holding Christina's hand in a hospital waiting room. That *is* my world. And changing it—even just a little—matters more than anything I could have done on a larger stage.

That one question reframed everything. It wasn't about legacy or big gestures or global impact. It was about how I could show up for the people I love. How I could leave joy in my wake. How I could make *my* world—my home, my family, my days—better, even if my body wasn't cooperating.

That conversation changed the way I think. The way I love.

The way I live.

And slowly, as my mental health improved, I noticed something else—my physical health did too. I had more energy. I smiled more. I moved more. I connected more. The weight started to lift. Not all at once, but steadily. Steadily enough to keep going.

All this from therapy.

So, if you're ever on the fence about getting help, I'll say this: don't wait until you hit bottom. Don't try to carry it all yourself. Even the strongest people need someone to talk to. Even those of us who pride ourselves on resilience need to unload the burden sometimes.

Therapy didn't fix everything. But it helped me see things differently. It gave me tools. It gave me words. And most importantly, it gave me *hope*.

Not just to exist—

But to *live*.

Therapy helped me untangle the knots in my mind, but what came next was a deeper transformation—the realization that I wasn't bound to the version of life I had lost. I could write something new. Not just survive—but actually reshape what life looked like from here.

CHAPTER 28: The Story I Thought I Was Writing

We all carry a story in our heads—a version of how life is supposed to go. A timeline. A map. A neat, linear plotline with chapter breaks and a satisfying ending.

For the first thirty-one years of my life, I thought I knew mine. I thought I knew the main characters. The pace. The themes. But what I've come to understand—through illness, distance, growth, and grief—is that sometimes life rips out the pages and hands you a blank one.

And when that happens, you only have two choices:

You can mourn the book you thought you were writing.

Or you can start a new one.

I didn't ask for cancer. I didn't plan for estrangement. I didn't build my dreams around pain, or surgeries, or staring down mortality at an age when most people are planning weekend barbecues.

But here we are.

I used to waste so much energy trying to get back to the story I thought I was supposed to be in. Trying to make it look *normal*. Trying to restore what was never coming back.

I told myself, *"Once I'm healthy again, things can go back to how they were."*

But the truth is, they never go back. And maybe that's not the worst thing.

At some point, I had to give myself permission to stop trying to return to a life that no longer fit.

I had to start asking different questions:

"What if this version of me—the one scarred, slower, softer—is still worth something?"

"What if the new life I build from here matters just as much as the one I lost?"

"What if the best chapters weren't at the beginning?"

Letting go of the old narrative wasn't easy. It felt like giving up at first. But it wasn't surrender. It was survival. And eventually, it became something more than that. It became liberation.

Maybe the story I was writing before was about achievement. Or recognition. Or proving something to the world.

The one I'm writing now?

It's about presence.

It's about small victories.

It's about making dinner with Christina and laughing with the kids and holding onto joy like it's a lifeline.

I used to think my legacy would be something big. Something bold. But now I realize it's quieter. It's in the way my daughter hugs her mom. It's in the way Jacob leads with patience. It's in the way Alex never lets a day pass without a joke.

The ending I imagined—the one I worked so hard for—isn't the one I'm getting.

But I'm starting to believe that this ending, the one I'm living now, might matter more than any version I once had in mind.

If you're reading this and you feel like your life has drifted too far from the shore—like the plot has gone off the rails—I hope you know this:

You're allowed to rewrite the story.

Even if it's halfway through.

Even if the ink has dried.

You don't need anyone else's permission.

You don't need a reason that satisfies everyone else.

You just need the courage to turn the page.

There are still days when I grieve the story I lost. Days when I look back and wonder, *"What if."*

But most days now, I look forward.

Because the story I'm writing—with Christina, with my kids, with this book—isn't one I ever planned for. But it's honest. It's hard. It's full of pain and laughter and growth and failure and forgiveness and grace.

And maybe, just maybe, that's the kind of story worth telling.

Of course, writing a new story doesn't mean forgetting the old one. Some chapters still haunt me—especially the ones that end with words left unsaid or relationships that couldn't be saved. But if rewriting is about reclaiming your life, forgiveness is about reclaiming your peace.

CHAPTER 29: Forgiving Us All

The lives we lead—full of decisions, detours, and defining moments—almost always leave behind traces of guilt, regret, or resentment. Sometimes we carry those feelings like a sharp needle tucked in our pocket: small, but always capable of piercing through when we least expect it. We convince ourselves it's manageable—even justified—but eventually, the weight becomes too much.

Not long ago, I was talking with a friend about this very thing. He said something that stopped me in my tracks:

"Resentment is drinking poison and expecting the other person to feel the pain. It only hurts us—the other person probably has no idea."

That hit me.

Because he was right—all that heaviness I'd carried around wasn't serving me. If anything, it was holding me back. Hearing it laid out so plainly made forgiveness feel less like giving something up and more like finally setting something down. And when you reframe it that way, forgiveness doesn't feel so impossible anymore. It starts to look like freedom.

There's also this idea that forgiveness is something you exclusively do for other people. A gift you offer to someone who hurt you. A bridge you build so you don't have to carry the weight of resentment anymore.

But the longer I live—and the closer I get to the edge of whatever's next—the more I've realized that the hardest forgiveness to give is often the kind that never leaves your own head. The kind you must give yourself.

And let's be honest: most of us are terrible at it.

Forgiving the Ones Who Couldn't Show Up

For a long time, I carried anger toward people who let me down—especially family. The ones who should've known better. The ones who should have been there.

It's a strange kind of pain when the people who gave you life become the source of so much hurt. And while the distance may have started with them, the choice to stay away eventually became mine. I've played that dance in my head over and over—asking what I could've done differently. How I might have made things easier. Whether it's too late now.

And maybe it is.

But I've learned that forgiveness doesn't mean reconciliation. It doesn't mean opening the door back up. Sometimes it just means saying:

"I no longer want this pain to own me."

It's not about absolving them. It's about unburdening yourself.

Forgiving Me

This part is the hardest.

I've had to forgive myself for all the things I couldn't prevent. For how long it took me to open my eyes. For how many years I went emotionally distant. For not always being the father, husband, or brother I should've been.

There were days—more than I'd like to admit—where I convinced myself that the world would go on just fine without me. That my family would recover. That my exit wouldn't really matter. But that wasn't true.

What I've come to understand—through therapy, reflection, and the steady love of the people closest to me—is that *presence* matters more than perfection. Just being here, being honest, being real—it's enough.

Forgiving myself didn't happen all at once. It still doesn't happen every day. But the more grace I extend to myself, the more I realize how much I've still got to give.

The Daily Practice of Grace

Forgiveness isn't a one-time event. It's a daily practice. A conscious decision to drop the weight you're carrying—even if only for a little while.

Some days I can't. I still pick it back up. I still replay things I wish I'd said. But more often now, I'm able to let it go.

Because at the end of the day, this life—this one wild, messy, beautiful life—is too short to keep bleeding from the same old wounds.

So, if you see yourself in these sentences, paragraphs, or pages, and you're holding on to something—some shame, some guilt, some ancient grudge—I hope you'll give yourself permission to let go. Or at least, to try.

Not because they deserve it. Maybe they don't.

But because *you* do.

Because you deserve peace.

Because you've already carried this long enough.

I've come to believe that forgiveness is a kind of quiet strength—one that softens the sharp edges of our past and makes space for something better. And as I've begun to forgive others, and slowly myself, I've started to see the ripple effects in unexpected places. In the way I parent. In how I show up for the people I love. And maybe most powerfully—in the way I remember the people who shaped me. Especially the ones who are no longer here.

Because not every relationship ends with closure. Not every goodbye is clean. But sometimes, the act of remembering—really remembering—is its own kind of forgiveness. Its own kind of love.

And that brings me to my dad.

CHAPTER 30: The Quiet Goodbye

It's strange how grief works. You expect it to hit all at once, to knock you down and keep you there. But sometimes, it arrives quietly—tucked inside old photos, or the way your son smiles just like your dad used to. For me, losing my father wasn't just about mourning the man he became at the end. It was about honoring the man he had always been—especially to me. Our story wasn't perfect, but it was ours. And it shaped me in more ways than I understood at the time.

When my dad died, it was a strange kind of heartbreak.

I cried. I mourned. I felt that familiar ache of loss. But just as much, I found myself replaying the good times—the memories that had shaped me more than I ever realized. The early evening runs. The family vacations packed into motorhomes. The long shifts at the gas station where I stood beside him, learning more about life than I did from most classrooms.

He and I built a bond that wasn't just father and son—it was built on time, on consistency, on trust. I was closer to him than my older siblings, not because he loved me more, but because we had *time* together. Shared routines. Shared jokes. Shared stubbornness.

And those blue eyes? I'm the only one who inherited them. A small thing, maybe. But it feels like proof that a piece of him lives on in me.

In the days following his death, I realized something I hadn't said often enough while he was alive: I truly loved him. Deeply. And his fingerprints are all over the kind of father I am today. The way I talk to my kids, the way I show up for them, the way I try to fix everything even when I can't—that all comes from him.

But it hurts to admit that my dad's story didn't end the way he probably imagined it would. His life, like so many, got sidetracked by stress, by a crumbling relationship with my mom, by disappointments and disease. Dementia crept in and stole pieces of him before we were ready to let go.

Toward the end, he wasn't the same man I remembered. He was smaller, frailer—a shell of the strong, clever, generous father I grew up idolizing. And visiting him during those final months was emotionally brutal. I had only a few chances to see him before he passed, and even fewer moments where I felt like *he* was still in there.

But there was one moment I'll never forget.

I went with my sister Kelly to visit him at the government care facility where he'd been living out his final time on this earth. She warned me before we went inside: that the conditions weren't great, that the place might smell, that the man I'd find might not recognize me at all. Dementia had fully taken hold. And it had been a long time since I'd seen him.

She told me not to be disappointed if I had to introduce myself like a stranger.

When we got there, he was asleep; something we were told he had been doing most of the day. It took nearly 15 minutes to wake him up. Eventually, he stirred and climbed slowly into his wheelchair. He looked at us blankly, like we were visitors from some forgotten part of his past. Kelly leaned forward, gently said hello again, trying to spark something in him.

And then she said, *"Look who's here."*

He looked up.

He stared directly into my eyes—and with a faint, almost broken smile, he said, *"Hey, Matt."*

My eyes filled instantly. I couldn't stop the tears.

Even if only for that one moment, he *saw* me. The way he used to. And that would be the last time I'd ever see him alive.

If that was to be the final memory of the man who taught me how to shoot a basketball, how to change the oil in my car, how to love and be loved… then honestly, I couldn't ask for a more perfect ending.

These days, I still see pictures of him from time to time. And I smile. I remember how much he adored Christina, how proud he was of my kids, how loudly he cheered for me in ways only a father can. I just hope they all know—my wife, my children—how lucky we were to have had him in our lives, even if for too short a time.

He was a great man. A man of faith. A man who gave more than he got. He wasn't big on speeches—he showed up early, stayed late, and said goodbye from the driveway with one hand already on the car door. And for all of that, I really do hope that there's something after this life—not just for his sake, but for all of ours. A place where sickness is gone. Where drama and disappointment fade. Where the only things left are the memories that matter. The laughter. The love. The second chances.

Because I'd give anything for just one more chance to look into those blue eyes and say what I didn't say enough while he was here:

"I love you, Dad."

You were everything I could have asked for.

In the silence that followed my father's passing, I was left with more than memories—I was left with echoes. Echoes of his voice, his laugh, his lessons. Some still bring comfort. Others still make me ache. But even in his absence, I find him everywhere—in my reflection, in my parenting, in the way I try to carry myself through life's heaviest moments. His love wasn't always loud, but it was steady. And now, it lives on in the way I love my own family—not perfectly, but fully.

There's one person who's felt the full weight of that love—and the full weight of the struggle that's come with it. The person who's stayed closest, stood strongest, and suffered most quietly. This final chapter is about her. About us.

CHAPTER 31: Burned and Bonded

People say that marriage is for better or worse, in sickness and in health. But they rarely explain what "worse" really looks like—or how long "sickness" can last. They don't tell you how hard it is to hold onto each other when everything around you is falling apart. Or how easy it is to forget who you are as a couple when all your energy goes toward simply surviving.

Christina and I have been through the fire—multiple times. We've stood on the edge of terrifying news. We've looked into the eyes of each other and wondered: *"Will we get through this? Will we be okay? Will I still have you next year... next month... tomorrow?"*

But somehow, we've always come back to each other.

When you're dealing with a life-altering illness, every conversation changes. Every plan comes with an asterisk. You're not just partners anymore—you're caregivers, co-survivors, emotional shock absorbers. The pressure builds quickly. You're exhausted and scared. One wrong word can feel like betrayal. One bad day can feel like everything's unraveling.

And still, the laundry needs folding. The kids need rides. The lawn needs to be mowed. It's all happening at once—the terrifying and the mundane—and through it all, your marriage is supposed to keep standing.

I'll be honest: it's not always graceful. There were those times I shut down emotionally. Times when I wasn't the husband Christina deserved. Times I let the weight of my own fear make me cold or distant. But the remarkable thing is—she never walked away from the fire. She stayed. She burned with me. And we kept finding each other in the flames.

Marriage during crisis demands a new kind of communication. It's not always about words. Sometimes it's a hand on your back during chemo. Sometimes it's knowing when *not* to talk. Sometimes it's crying at the same time, and sometimes it's taking turns so the other one can fall apart first.

There are days when we argue—not because we didn't love each other, but because grief is messy. Fear can make you short-tempered. Pain can make you selfish. But at the end of it all, we keep choosing each other. Even on the worst days. Especially on the worst days.

And I learned—slowly, but surely—how to love her better through all of it. Not with grand gestures, but with presence. With humility. With apologies. With reminders that she was not just my caregiver, but still my partner, my friend, my girl.

No one talks enough about what happens to intimacy in the middle of trauma. It doesn't disappear, but it changes shape. Sometimes it's holding hands in a waiting room. Sometimes it's laughing together in the middle of chaos. Sometimes it's a text that says, *"I'm thinking of you,"* even when you're in the same room.

There's a tenderness that gets forged when you've seen each other at rock bottom. I've seen her cry through pain. She's seen me break down in fear. And through that shared exposure— that raw, stripped-back honesty—something deeper emerged. A love that's been tested. Weathered. Proven.

Looking back now, I don't think the fire tested our marriage. I think it refined it.

We've grown. We've failed and forgiven. We've had to say *"I'm sorry"* more times than I can count, and *"I love you"* even more. And somehow, through it all, we've found a version of love that is deeper, more honest, and more sacred than I ever thought possible.

If you are walking through your own version of the fire—I won't tell you it's easy. It's not. But I will tell you this:

Hold on.

Let the fire burn away what doesn't matter. Let it draw you closer, not further apart. Let it show you what love looks like when everything else fades away.

Because that love? That's the kind that survives anything.

We've come to understand that the strongest acts of love are rarely loud. They're almost always quiet, persistent, and often go unnoticed. But every now and then, love calls for a moment—one that stands out, not because it's showy, but because it's redemptive. A moment that rewrites regret and transforms pain into something beautiful.

And as it turns out, I had one of those moments in me after all…

One of the biggest regrets I carried for years—and something Christina would good-naturedly tease me about from time to time—was breaking up with her early in our relationship and missing her senior prom. We still found our way back to each other, but that gap in time left a void I always wished I could fill. After my second diagnosis, during one of our darker periods filled with worry and stress, I started thinking of ways to bring back joy. Something unexpected. Something healing. Something just for her.

So, I did the only logical thing you can think of for your 25th Anniversary: I threw a surprise prom. A 1993-themed prom, no less.

With the help of a small army of friends and family, I secretly booked a local community center that looked like a high school gym. I sent out invites to over 150 people. I even got Tim and Karie to fly in from Colorado. Olivia helped me find a dress that closely resembled the one Christina wore to her real prom. And I tracked down the baggiest tuxedo I could find to match the era.

The night before the big event, I snuck out the basement door, changed into a vintage '90s outfit, crept around the side of the house, and rang the doorbell. When Christina opened the door, she saw me holding a sign that read:

"You can't simply turn back the hands of time, just to relive one night,

but let's pretend it's 1993 so I can make my wrong a right! PROM?"

Thankfully, she said yes.

And since I was the one organizing the whole thing—let's just say the vote for prom king and queen may have been slightly influenced in our favor.

The night was perfect. A DJ played our throwback playlist. Friends arrived dressed in retro formalwear. The decorations screamed high school nostalgia. Even the non-alcoholic punch may have been "inadvertently" spiked. But what made it unforgettable was the joy on Christina's face—a mixture of surprise, laughter, and that quiet understanding we share when words aren't even necessary.

It was silly and over the top. And it was absolutely worth it.

We'll never forget that night. Not because of the music or

the lights or even the hilarity of watching grown adults re-live their teenage years—but because it was a moment of lightness in a stretch of life that had grown so heavy. It was my way of rewriting one of my oldest mistakes and reminding Christina that even after 25 years, there's still magic to be made.

Life doesn't always give you do-overs. You don't often get the chance to revise history, fix a regret, or go back and make something right. But every once in a while, if you're lucky—*really* lucky—you get to step back into a moment you thought had passed you by. You get to say, *"This time, I'm showing up."*

That's what that night was for me. For us.

It wasn't just a prom. It wasn't just a tux or a rented room, or a cheesy sign taped to a foam board. It was a symbol. That no matter what life has thrown our way—illness, loss, uncertainty, mistakes—we've always found a way back to each other. Back to love. Back to joy.

We danced that night like kids who had no clue what was ahead of them. And in some ways, we *were* those kids. Just older now. Wiser. Grayer (well, one of us). But still full of the same magic that's carried us through it all.

These moments are essential to keep some semblance of sanity because at the end of the day, this awful disease is constantly lurking, ready to bring a level of destruction to those joyous flashes. Reality always finds a way of creeping back in, and the cycle starts all over again.

Cancer has taken a lot from me—my health, my comfort, my confidence, my ability to plan for the future without holding my breath. But some of its cruelest wounds aren't the visible ones. Some of the hardest battles take place not in hospital rooms or scan reports, but in the quiet spaces between people who love each other.

I've written a lot about Christina—the way we've leaned on one another, laughed through tears, found strength in partnership. And all of that is true. But it's not the whole truth. The whole truth is harder. The whole truth is that even in the strongest relationships, cancer doesn't just hit one person—it hits both people. It hits the whole house. And sometimes it leaves cracks that love alone can't immediately patch.

There are many days when I feel like I'm the reason for all of this—the stress, the sadness, the uncertainty. I didn't choose to have cancer, but I am undeniably the source of it in our lives. That guilt is heavy. Even when I know better, it still lingers— like background noise I can't turn off. I carry a constant ache knowing that Christina's life would be easier—freer—if she hadn't married a man with a body full of bad news.

There are moments when I wonder if she resents me. I don't think she does, not really—not in a deep, abiding way. But resentment has a sneaky way of slipping in through exhaustion, fear, and heartbreak. Maybe it's not even resentment toward me, but toward the whole situation. Toward the fact that our life together has been so weighted by appointments and medications and waiting rooms. Toward the quiet envy of people who get to plan carefree weekends or spontaneous getaways—people who don't live with a cloud hanging over them. And I get it. Sometimes I envy them too.

Sometimes I wonder if she's still in love with me. Not "love"—I never question that. She's proven it, repeatedly. But "in love" is different. "In love" means you still get butterflies. It means you look across the room and smile just because. It means wanting to reach for each other instead of just reaching for the calendar to see when the next treatment is. I know we're still in this together. I know she's still here. But there are days when the spark feels buried under the weight of everything else.

There are times when it feels like we're just coexisting—living side by side, but not exactly together. When I'm not feeling well—which is often—I go into a kind of protective mode. I shut down, not because I don't want to connect, but because I don't want to burden anyone. I don't want to look into her eyes and see her worry reflected back at me. I convince myself that bottling it up is my way of shielding her. But silence can be just as loud as pain. And in those quiet spells, she retreats too. She gets short-tempered and distant. I can feel her frustration. I can feel her fear. And neither of us has the words to break through it.

We always find our way back. That's the beautiful part. We snap out of it eventually. But these episodes—they happen more than they used to. It's a cycle we never imagined we'd be in, and we don't always know how to break it. Cancer doesn't just test your body. It tests your love. It stretches the seams of your relationship and demands that you keep choosing each other, even when the road feels joyless.

People often focus on the physical toll cancer takes—the surgeries, the fatigue, the scans. But the emotional toll is heavier, and it's harder to talk about. The physical pain you can treat. You can measure it. You can name it. But the emotional pain? The doubt, the distance, the guilt, the quiet resentment—it's harder to name. And even harder to heal.

But I believe that naming it is part of the healing. And if you're reading this, and you've felt any version of what I'm describing, I want you to know this: You're not failing. You're not alone. Even strong marriages bend under this kind of pressure. But bending doesn't mean breaking.

We're still here. Still holding on. Still choosing each other. Even in the silence. Even in the hard parts. Especially in the hard parts.

Even on the toughest days, when we're distant or discouraged or worn out from the weight of it all, we always come back to the same truth: love brought us here, and love is what keeps us here.

It doesn't always look romantic. Sometimes love is quiet— a gentle touch when you're not speaking, or a partner who remembers your next scan even when you don't. Sometimes it's showing up when it's hard. Sometimes it's staying when you want to run. And sometimes, it's simply continuing to choose each other in the middle of all this mess.

I may never be able to give Christina the life she dreamed of, free from hospitals and prescriptions and hard conversations. But I can give her this: my presence. My effort. My love. And on most days, that still feels like enough.

I don't know how much time I have left. But I know this: I've lived a full life. I've loved deeply. I've messed up. I've made amends. I've laughed until my ribs hurt and cried until my heart broke. And somehow, I've kept going.

Not every chapter ended the way I thought it would. Some relationships faded. Some bridges burned. But the ones that stayed? They shine brighter than ever.

So, if this is the last chapter—and who knows if it is—let it end the way every good story should.

With music playing.

With friends by your side.

With the love of your life in your arms.

And with your feet still moving.

Because even when the world tells you to sit this one out,

sometimes you just have to stand up, smile…

…and dance.

...

In the end, "normal" was never one fixed thing. It shifted with every chapter — from survival, to perspective, to peace. And maybe that's the point. A life worth living doesn't follow one definition. It writes its own.

EPILOGUE: In Their Words

I've spent this entire book telling my story through my eyes—the love I've felt, the pain I've endured, the moments that made me feel most alive. But I didn't live this life alone. I asked a few of the people who've been on this journey with me to share their perspectives—not to validate my story, but to expand it. What follows are their voices, their truths, their love—in their own words.

———————

My dad is the kind of person that everyone wants to be around. He's kind, funny, hardworking, and generous—the kind of man who will always put others before himself without ever expecting anything in return. He is the strongest guy I know, and his strength is what keeps our family's strength together. There's no better compliment than when someone tells me I have my dad's personality—it makes me proud to remind people of someone as amazing as him. The perfect depiction of who he is as a person was during his speech at my brother Alex's wedding. The way he had me, and everyone else, going from tears to laughs shows his warmth and humor all in one.

He's not just my dad—he's truly my best friend. He's someone I know I can always count on for advice, to always be there for me, and of course a laugh. He truly is the funniest person I know and will always know how to put a smile on my face. I'm forever going to advocate that we start our father-daughter stand-up comedy act! I feel blessed to be able to call him my dad and can never thank him enough for everything he has done for me in my life and continues to do each day.

My dad is the person I could sit and listen to all day long, whether it's stories about his childhood, his college years, or the other random memories that come to his mind. He's also my go-to person for everything and anything – whether he always likes it or not. I'll have him on speed dial with all IT questions, usually something about my car, or when I'm looking for movie and TV show recommendations.

Something I will never forget and will always hold close to my heart is our father-daughter dances. Even though we liked to master the beginning of the dance before moving our way to the back, nothing can replace how special it was to get to share the stage with him every year. It's one of the top things I look forward to doing on my wedding day – we should be pros; we did it for 10 years! Having him on the sidelines cheering on each and every volleyball game made each play feel even more meaningful knowing I had him and my mom supporting me every second of the way. I'll always remember my favorite season of volleyball to be the one where my parents stepped up to coach my fifth-grade team. Being able to share the game I loved with the two people I loved the most was something I will forever cherish.

I'll always be grateful that we both went to the University of Wisconsin. It feels so special to have been able to walk the same campus and experience the same things he did during his college years. I'll never forget how memorable he made my first day at UW, when he snuck on my phone and added Rascal

Flatts, *My Wish* and then sent me a text as he drove away from school telling me to listen to the last song added on my phone. Something so small that I've held on to all these years and will forever think of him and that moment when I hear that song.

He always knows exactly what to say, especially in all of life's biggest moments. His words always make me feel so loved, proud, and special as his daughter. I easily speak for everyone when I say to know him is to love him.

And to you Dad, I hope you always know how much you mean to me. You've always been my biggest supporter and my favorite person to laugh with. You've shown me what real strength, loyalty, and love look like through everything you do every single day. You have taught me what it means to be a good person, a great friend, a sports lover, and you have no question set the highest bar for what I look for in a man. I hope to find someone as kind, respectful, thoughtful, and loving as you are to mom and us kids.

I am proud of you each and every day for your perseverance and continual ability to be strong through everything life has thrown at you. Your strength, determination, and dedication in everything you do continues to inspire me every day to work harder and be better. You never fail to surprise me with your next aspiration you set your mind to.

Thank you for being the kind of dad who I can also call my best friend. Thank you for all the sacrifices you've made, for the way you love our family, and for always being someone I can count on. I am so grateful to be your daughter, and I hope you know that you've shaped me into the person I am today. I work every day hoping to make you proud, because everything that I am is a reflection of the way you've raised me. I'll always be a daddy's girl and will forever be your little

Boo.

I love you, Dad—more than I could ever put into words.

Olivia

Dad,

To say I have been lucky to have grown up with you as my father is an understatement; I have been truly blessed. I have had the best role model my whole life to show me how to be a real man. You have been the most caring and selfless individual I know, genuinely caring for all. Everything you do is for our family, and I hope I can emulate that as my life goes on. I have always admired your way of parenting; you are more than just a father; you've been a great friend. At any given moment you're there for me. Anything from life advice in a stressful time or to just watching a game with me, you're always there. I am glad we can be such great friends. I don't think many others could say the same about their parents, so I am grateful. No matter what is going on in my life, I know I can count on you, I don't know what I would do without you. Through and through, you have been a best friend and an amazing father.

Through the past nearly 10 years, you've had to go through hell. With this ongoing cancer battle, your strength and patience have taught me so much. Despite the difficult days and seemingly never-ending fight, you put on a smile every day and continue to be there for me and our whole family. I will forever admire your strength to get through each day, treatment, and surgery. Maybe it's just the dad strength, but you really are stronger than I could ever be. As the fight continues, I will forever be by your side until you finally kick cancer's ass. I don't take a single day with you for granted, each day is a blessing, and I am always excited for the next.

One positive to come out of this whole situation is what you have taught me about life. You have made it clear to me that the single most important thing in life is happiness. You continue to live your life to the fullest despite the setbacks, and that has shown me what I need to do. No matter the situation, you have helped me realize I need to prioritize what will make me happy, without having to always worry about silly consequences like missing a class or spending a bit too much money. This has allowed me to experience so much more in life and break out of my comfort zone a bit. You may not have even realized that you made this impact on me, but I have known and I am so grateful for it. Just having seen how you live life and moving to Florida with you has made me so happy and guided my life in the right direction. Thank you.

Some of my favorite memories with you have already come from this short time in Florida together. One example has been going to the USF basketball and football games with you. A major reason why I decided to go to USF was to be at the closest school to you, and to be able to share a part of my college experience with you has been amazing. Getting to sit in the stands with you and talk about the USF teams all through their ups and downs has been the best. It is so relaxing to just not have to think about anything else and enjoy the game with you. It truly has been a special bonding moment for me, and I hope you know that. It has brought us closer together, and I will never forget these memories. And you always fit right in with the rest of the students in the student section!

Finally, I just want to thank you again for everything. Thank you for being who you are. Thank you for being an amazing friend and father; and thank you for giving me these great looks! As I grow up, I will strive to be as great of a father as you have been. I hope to continue to live life like you and appreciate it as much as you do. You will never fully know how much I try to be just like you. Thank you for everything.

I love you,

Jake

I am so proud of my dad, and I am honored to be able to add something to this book. That said, I'm not usually a very serious writer so I'll share a story that I think describes our family well, especially our ability to find the humor in everything.

When my grandpa passed away a few years ago, the funeral was the first time the whole extended family was all in the same place, at the same time in more than a decade. This day wasn't about any of that though, it was about celebrating and honoring a great man. Despite its sadness and the freezing winter temperatures, the day was beautiful. To cap off the ceremony, Uncle Andrew performed with a two-person band to sing an Irish Blessing my grandpa loved. Now, no matter what, Andrew has always been the comic relief in our lives, and it's never because we are making fun of him, but always because we love him and because he has always been such a joy to be around. He is hilarious whether he is trying to be or not. Well anyways, to cap a nice ceremony the two members of the band were outperformed by Andrew's loud singing masking their gentle singing. Full disclosure...Andrew isn't a great singer (not that I have any room to talk), but you have to admire how loudly and proudly he sings at church. At first, it gave me a small chuckle because like I said, growing up with Andrew, seeing him as a big brother at times, and then as I got older hearing stories about him as a kid, things like him singing loudly and off pitch make me chuckle. But then my brief smile and chuckle turned into full-blown-crying-laughter as Andrew decided to start boisterously serenading his brother's wife (AKA my mom) from across the church, loudly professing into the microphone *"I love you Chrissie Arnold"* and *"I'm coming over to your house every day"* as the band tried desperately to hold their notes and lyrics. Unfortunately, my dad's attempts to sternly and silently get him to stop only egged him on more, as those things always did. When the song (finally) ended, the priest said *"Thank you, Andrew"* which made me laugh even harder. It's extra funny because I don't think many outside of close family were laughing. Now, for some families this may have ruined the ceremony. But if one thing is certain, we are not just "some family." Being able to have Andrew make us laugh so hard, especially now looking back at it, is a memory that I, and I think all of us, will forever cherish as something honestly deeper than it really was. Andrew has always been everyone's favorite since he always knows how to make everyone's day better.

To be more candid than telling a silly story, and I've said this before, if anyone can beat cancer again, it's my dad. He fights so hard and has such a positive attitude about it and I am so proud. You may not even know talking to him that he's sick.

Thanks for letting me add a story I think about often to this book!

Alex

—————————

I don't remember the exact moment I met Saunders over 20 years ago—but I'll never forget how he made me feel. His warmth wrapped around me like a favorite, well-worn sweatshirt. He listened—really listened—with a genuine interest that made me feel seen, heard, and valued. That's just who he is. Anyone lucky enough to be in his orbit feels important. Conversations with Saunders don't just go in one ear and out the other; they stick. He remembers things—not just the big moments, but the small, quiet details too. And he asks about them later, giving them—and you—meaning.

If you haven't figured it out by now, Saunders is known for his killer sense of humor: quick, dry, and brilliantly smart. He has a gift for turning everyday life into stand-up comedy, delivering punchlines with perfect timing. If you need proof, watch the speech he gave at his son Alex's wedding—it should be a Netflix-special. Humor has always been his superpower, his way of coping even when life got hard. I've admired that about him deeply, wishing I could channel that same resilience.

But there were two moments when that humor didn't show up—both times when he told me about his cancer diagnosis. I waited for the joke, the zinger, the classic Saunders twist. But it never came. And that silence said everything. I saw my friend overwhelmed, vulnerable, hurting. It shattered me. Because bad things shouldn't happen to people like Saunders - people who love so selflessly and fiercely. People who live to protect and keep those they love free from pain.

I've never seen anyone care so deeply for the people in their life. Saunders carries the weight of others' heartache, always trying to shield his loved ones from what hurts. I have countless examples of this from over the years. Cancer stole that from him. It robbed him of the ability to protect in the way he always had. And I hate cancer for that. I can only imagine the pain it's caused him, it kills me knowing how much he struggles with that loss. More than anything, I wish I could take the pain away. I wish I could give him back the ability to protect the people he loves. But I can't. None of us can.

What I can do is carry his legacy forward. I can love harder. I can show up more. I can make damn sure the people in my life know they are safe, valued and deeply loved – always. I can fight to be selfless in my love, just like he's always done, even when it comes at a price.

I've always cherished my friendship with Saunders. Having him in my life is one of my greatest gifts. The way he lives – with courage, humor and heart, even in the face of death, is a masterclass in what it means to be human. It's a lesson I'll carry with me for the rest of my life. And one I'll keep learning, every single day.

I love you, Saunders. Thank you for being such an important part of my life.

Elke

—————————

I have many memories of my time with my Uncle Matt, but probably some of my finest are our trips to his house in Sussex. I loved the long drive and anticipation that took us to his house, and I love the greeting I received. *"Hi, Ellabear!"* Uncle Matt would shout. I would run to his arms, and he would pick me up. *"What's up, EB?"* he would say, another abbreviation for Ellabear. I reveled in his attention, especially when my brother,

Seamus, came along. I will always treasure my trips and the nicknames from Uncle Matt, the smell of his house and garage, the comfy couch, and the warm hugs that started and ended every one of our visits.

Ella

———————

Hey Matt,

We're not going to say too many nice things about you here because we don't want you to get a fat head (JK). We can already just imagine you saying, *"but I already have a fat head!"* That's a simple example of your often self-deprecating humor. Humor is probably one of the first things that we loved about you. You've always been so incredibly quick-witted and entertaining. Way back when you were only seventeen and began dating our daughter, is when we began enjoying you and your outgoing personality. Thirty-four years later, although so much has happened and changed, our love for you and your persona has only grown.

Speaking about seventeen-year-olds, it seems Christina was only seventeen and you were eighteen at the time that we may have had at least one concern about you dating our daughter. If we said nothing more about that here, you would still know exactly what we're about to mention. That's right—the family camping trip you joined us on, the beer that you had procured, and a trip to the Vilas County courthouse. As you know, we were less than thrilled about that whole thing, but especially since Christina's court-ordered punishment became **our** punishment! Since she was not allowed to drive for a while, it meant that **we** had to be her chauffeur for work, school, appointments, etc.! You may still owe for that fiasco. Fortunately, you must have groveled enough, and we didn't hold a grudge. Admittedly, we do like hearing you describe how we made you come along to the courthouse with us and how you felt like that was the longest car ride **ever**.

The next five years flew by (as usual) and we had so many more fun times with you and Christina that by the time you two got married, we were absolutely thrilled to have you become our son-in-law. Yes, we were turning our oldest child over to you and that was a little scary. Not because it was you Matt, it could have been anyone, even some wealthy or super smart guy! But thinking back to that day, the look and constant smile on Christina's face said it all. There was no doubt in our minds that you made her happy. Of course, that made us happy. You have proven in the past 28 years that you continue to make her happy. You've been a fantastic husband, an awesome father, and a terrific and loveable son to us.

We would have to write an entire book here to cover all the great times we've enjoyed together, but certainly the most joyous were when you and Christina gave us our three oldest grandchildren. The joy continued as we were included in so many birthdays, holidays, graduations, dance recitals, baseball games, basketball games, volleyball games, camping trips, Florida and Disney World trips, up north and other vacations, and family gatherings. We thank God every day for family!

Unfortunately, we've had some very sad times in our family too. Some of the saddest was your cancer diagnosis on multiple occasions. Each time, the news was like daggers to our hearts. And of course, the surgeries and treatments and on going suffering continue to bring tears to our eyes even if we don't always show it. Nobody can explain why some good people must endure sickness or disease. Only God knows. We do know that God does not control these things on earth, but He simply allows nature to take whatever course it happens to take and allows people to make good or bad choices. You have made an outstanding choice to persevere and battle your cancer in every way you can. You've made an outstanding choice to be strong for your family who love you so dearly and whom you love so dearly. We know that far too frequently, this must be unbearably difficult for you. You have our endless admiration for how you have handled this burden, and can only encourage you to keep fighting!

It seems that when dealing with cancer, even words of encouragement bring a level of sadness, so let's change the subject. Do you remember all these far less serious things:

- When, during the night on a camping trip, an unravelling hose in a bucket caused you to freak out that some unknown critter was nearby?
- When you accidentally squished a bullfrog while wearing soccer sandals while visiting the outhouse?
- When you drove out of the campground in your dad's motor home and smacked off the antenna that you forgot to lower?
- When you tied up the canoe so poorly that the mooring rope unraveled as soon as your poor father-in-law stepped in and immediately plunged into the lake?
- The countless times you slammed your head on something (usually due to a baseball cap brim blocking your vision)?
- Tricking your 5-year-old daughter Olivia, who knew letters but could not actually read, into writing *"I am a chicken and I wear diapers"* when she had asked for help in

writing a nice note to her teacher?

- How you continually played catcher for Alex as he practiced baseball pitching in your yard even though he nearly broke your thumb or finger?
- How you pushed your little nephew Calvin in his go-cart so far and fast down the driveway that he ran away in disgust yelling *"I told you I didn't want to go that **stupid** far!"*?
- On numerous occasions, encouraging little Cal to do all sorts of crazy things like break dancing or running wildly from an imaginary mountain lion you assured him was lurking around?
- Over the years, encouraging all of your nephews and nieces (when they were little) to do or say anything that might embarrass their parents or themselves?

Matt, you are one of a kind and we have been so blessed to have you in our lives and our family. We love you more than you may know!

Sincerely,
Tom and Patty
(Dad and Mom)

Author's Note...

Before you read Christina's words, I want to be very clear about something.

Asking her to contribute to this book was not a simple request. She has carried more of this story than anyone else—often silently, often without recognition—and much of what she has endured lives far beyond what words can capture.

She wrestled with whether to write anything at all. Not because she had nothing to say, but because some experiences don't belong to explanation. They belong to survival. To presence. To love shown in ways that don't need translation.

What she chose to share is brief by design. It is not incomplete. It is not careful. It is enough. It reflects the strength, restraint, and honesty that have defined her throughout this journey.

I ask that her words be received as they are—without expectation, without interpretation, and without judgment. They are offered in love, and in trust.

I am grateful beyond measure that she chose to share even this small part of herself. It is a gift I will always protect.

Matt,

I truly can't remember my life before you and I can't imagine it without you. I love the life we've created together, especially our three amazing kids who mean the world to me. However, the journey hasn't been easy and watching you battle cancer now for 10 years has broken my heart. I wish you could be healthy again and go back to living a normal life, although I don't even remember what that is like anymore. People tell me I'm strong, but I feel weak because I can't do anything to make you better. No matter what, I will always be by your side doing the best I can to support you. I'm so grateful to have the best husband who always puts me first. With all that you've been through it amazes me how you are always more concerned about how I am. I love you so much!

Christina

These aren't just people I love—they're the chapters of my life I couldn't write alone. If I've learned anything from all of this, it's that we are never remembered for our pain, or even our accomplishments, but by the people who carry our stories forward.